Sardinia's Fountain of Youth

A Journey into the Blue Zones

by Francis Domenico

Formatted, Converted, and Distributed by eBookIt.com
http://www.eBookIt.com

ISBN-13: 9781456641979 (paperback)
ISBN-13: 9781456641962 (ebook)
ISBN-13: 9781456641986 (audiobook)

Dear Esteemed Reader,

Thank you immensely for choosing this book to join your collection. We imagine that you've already embarked on an exploration of ideas within these pages, and we couldn't be happier about it!

Now, if you find yourself chuckling, pondering, or even debating with the words in front of you, we'd absolutely love to hear about it. If you can spare a few moments to pen down your thoughts in a review, we would be as delighted as a dictionary on a spelling bee!

An Amazon review would be excellent - but hey, we're far from picky. Whether it's a scribble on the back of a grocery list, a tweet, or even a message in a bottle (though that might take a while to reach us), your feedback is gold.

Writing a review might not be as fun as a spontaneous dance-off, but we promise it'll bring grins to our faces, warmth to our hearts, and incredibly valuable insights to future readers.

With Gratitude,

Bo Bennett, PhD
Publisher
Archieboy Holdings, LLC.

Table of Contents

Sardinia's Enigmatic Longevity

Enveloped in the azure expanses of the Mediterranean, rests an island with secrets of extraordinary longevity beguiling the globe. This is Sardinia, an alluring idyll where time appears in perpetual lull, and people's lifespans outdo those in most other regions. Among its rocky terrains and charming pastel-hued homes thrive a populace that embodies the essence of an authentic 'Blue Zone' — the world's rare locales that harbor an unusually high proportion of centenarians. While Blue Zones continue to baffle scientists worldwide, Sardinia stands as a beacon of unique intrigue. Key to Sardinia's fascinating longevity is a compelling medley of salubrious diet, robust social bonds, active and fulfilling lifestyle, and deeply ingrained cultural practices. Of course, it's a nuanced interplay of these several factors that contribute to the extended lifespans observed here. As we embark on this captivating journey, let's delve into Sardinia's enigmatic longevity secrets and decipher the formula for a longer, healthier life tucked in its winding cobblestoned alleys and sun-drenched landscapes.

The Mystery of the Blue Zones

In our quest for sustainable living and longevity, little is as intriguing as the phenomenon known as "Blue Zones." These are small geographic pockets scattered across the world where people live significantly longer than average. In these areas, it's not unusual to encounter octogenarians, nonagenarians, or even centenarians frequently.

The term 'Blue Zone' isn't one found in geography textbooks; instead, it's a concept coined by demographers, Gianni Pes, and Michel Poulain, working in conjunction with journalists, Dan Buettner. After observing an unusual concentration of centenarians in specific regions, they marked them in blue, thus leading to the term, 'Blue Zones.'

The idea encapsulates five regions globally: Okinawa in Japan, Nicoya in Costa Rica, Icaria in Greece, Loma Linda in California, and, the subject of this book, Sardinia in Italy. What makes these zones fascinating is not just the remarkably high age that many residents attain, but also their quality of life. Most individuals maintain physical and mental acuity, despite their advanced years, defying the traditional narrative surrounding aging.

Our focus will be Sardinia, an island region off Italy that is home to one of the oldest populations on the earth. The mountainous Barbagia region, in particular, boasts more than ten times the number of centenarians per capita than the US and thrice the Italian average.

This intriguing statistical anomaly has been the subject of several research projects and studies, seeking to unravel the secrets hidden within Sardinia's splendid landscapes. What differentiates Sardinia from the other 'Blue Zones', and thereby the rest of the world? What are the lifestyle and behavior patterns that set these residents apart, attributing to their health and longevity?

Regardless of the number of books and scholarly articles written about the Blue Zones, the reasons behind this unique longevity remain somewhat veiled in mystery. Diet, while crucial, can't be the only piece of the puzzle, considering the variety between the regions.

The isolation of Sardinia, for example, led to a distinct culinary evolution that gave rise to a Mediterranean diet rich in whole grains, fruits, vegetables, and healthy fats. Likewise, the other Blue Zones have established unique dietary habits formed by their geographical isolation and cultural roots.

Diet alone, however, isn't the key to understanding this phenomenon. The physical activities that constitute an integral part of daily life in these regions also play their part. In all the Blue Zones, locals lead active lives with regular, low-intensity physical activity like gardening, walking, or housework. But again, diet and exercise are factors universally acknowledged to contribute to long life. Hence, they can't be the sole reasons for such extraordinary longevity.

The Sardinian culture and its emphasis on strong familial ties, community involvement, and social engagement cannot be ignored either. The sense of belonging, shared history, and communal companionship have significant effects on the mental and emotional well-being of individuals, fostering a considerably more satisfying life.

Moreover, the Sardinians stress the art of savoring life, whether it's through slow, leisurely meals, sharing stories with loved ones, or simply basking in the gentle Mediterranean sun. This mindfulness approach, the ceaseless appreciation and enjoyment of each moment, has been suggested as an important contributor to their longevity.

The Sardinians' spiritual beliefs and practices also play a subtle yet significant role, offering solace, guidance, and tangible health benefits diminished stress levels. However, none of these factors seem to fully encapsulate the secrets held within Sardinia or the other Blue Zones.

So, the question remains: what is the secret sauce? Does it lie in some undisclosed lifestyle aspect indigenous to these regions? Or is it an intricate weaving of the factors already mentioned—diet, physical activity, socially engaging culture, appreciation for life, familial connections, and spiritual practices—that compile the chapters of life in a Blue Zone?

The Journey begins; we'll probe scientifically and anecdotally, diving into the Sardinian way of life with an open mind and curious spirit. The aim is to uncover ways an average person outside these zones can incorporate some of the 'Blue Zone magic' into their life, journeying towards longer, healthier living.

Unveiling the mysteries of Sardinia's longevity will be an exhilarating exploration, leading us on scenic trails laden with unexpected revelations and timeless wisdom. As we dispel the fog surrounding the Blue Zones, we'll uncover the complex interplay between individual behaviors, community dynamics, dietary practices, and the environment.

Sardinia's Place in the Longevity Landscape

Why is Sardinia unique amongst the world's longevity hotspots? What is it about this beautiful Mediterranean island that has allowed its people to claim one of the top spots in the global longevity rankings? To unravel Sardinia's secret to long life, we'll need to delve deeper into its idiosyncrasies while maintaining a broad perspective on the global longevity landscape.

It isn't solely the picturesque environment or even the area's distinctly Mediterranean climate that makes Sardinia special in the context of longevity. Other locales share similar characteristics. Tracing the Sardinian longevity phenomenon requires rich a tapestry of interconnected factors that interplay in the island's terrain.

The Blue Zones, areas of the world where individuals live significantly longer and healthier lives, are distributed across the globe. Besides Sardinia, these include Okinawa in Japan, Nicoya in Costa Rica, Ikaria in Greece, and Loma Linda in California. Each of these areas is unique, shaped by different historical, cultural, and environmental influences. Yet, they all share one commonality: an unusually high proportion of centenarians among their population.

Sardinia differs from its Blue Zone counterparts in its rich tapestry of lifestyle habits, diet, community, and overall approach to life that sets it apart. The island's strength lies in its ability to seamlessly integrate these elements to nurture a culture of longevity.

Remarkably, Sardinia holds the title of having the highest number of male centenarians in the world, a distinction which in other Blue Zones, women usually claim. This finding further underscores Sardinia's unique position within the longevity landscape.

The distinct geographical identification of Sardinia is another essential factor. Sardinia is more condensed and localized compared to other Blue Zones cultures, whose age-related outliers are spread across broader and more diverse regions. This high concentration gives scientists an ideal laboratory to study the conditions favorable to enduring vitality.

Additionally, the island's relative isolation through much of its history has created a genetic bottleneck, allowing the quality of long-lived genes to extend and multiply from one generation to another.

The longevity hotspots of Sardinia are concentrated in a region known as Barbagia. Interestingly, within the genetic hotbed of longevity genes, Barbagia stands out even further. The rugged, mountainous region has maintained a traditional lifestyle largely untouched by modern influences, thereby preserving age-old practices conducive to long life.

It's crucial to note that longevity in Sardinia is not merely about reaching a notable age but doing so while maintaining a high quality of life. Sardinians are not only long-lived but tend to enjoy exceptional health and vitality into the latter stages of life.

Far from being a mere statistical anomaly, Sardinia represents a living embodiment of healthy, active aging, where people retain their physical strength, mental clarity, and youthful spirit long into the twilight years. This aspect reinforces Sardinia's unique position in the global longevity landscape.

While every Blue Zone has valuable lessons about longevity to offer, Sardinia's uniqueness encompasses not merely its individuals' lifespans, but the quality of their long lives—well-lived, rich in tradition, family, and community relationships, mental balance, work, and a diet imbued with regional and seasonal foods. They're active both physically and socially, in touch with nature, and live their lives with purpose.

Taking a holistic view, the 'secrets' to Sardinian longevity are broadly woven into the island's community and culture, encompassing elements such as dietary habits, social engagement, physical activity, spirituality, strong familial ties, and a robust work ethic. The combination of these factors in a traditionally maintained setting is what makes Sardinia singular.

Researchers and thinkers across the globe continue to study Sardinia, looking to understand how to apply its lessons to improve health and longevity elsewhere. While it's important to remember that replicating Sardinia's success necessarily involves adapting to each unique context, Sardinia certainly serves as an inspiring model for an aging world.

In conclusion, Sardinia's place in the longevity landscape paints a vibrant picture of an island where life is lived fully and well past the usual lifespan. This region stands as a testament to living proof that not only can human beings live longer, but also that we can age with grace, vitality, and joyful engagement in life.

Overview of the Journey Ahead

We are on the brink of an intriguing exploration, a dive into the profound mystery of longevity housed in the charming lands of Sardinia. Did Sardinia stumble upon the fountain of youth or is there a method to this enchanting mystery? We seek answers as we embark on our journey to understand the phenomenon of the 'Blue Zones' and Sardinia's auspicious positioning within it.

Our journey through the realm of centenarians commences with a complete grasp of Sardinia's geographical and demographic landscape in the first chapter. Sardinia's unique historical background houses rich cultures intertwined with bits and pieces that play parts in its uncanny longevity.

Next, we take a gastronomic expedition into the Sardinian diet. The Mediterranean influences, the local ingredients, the ancient recipes – every aspect of their culinary world is a fragment of the riddle that is longevity. The connection between their diet and extended lifespan is an area of study that requires special attention.

We then investigate the incredibly tight-knit communal and familial fabric of Sardinia's population. Social engagement and mental health go hand in hand and unveil the potential role of strong social bonds and mental wellbeing in this exceptional lifespan.

In chapter four, we delve into their daily routines, patterning physical activity into lives. The intimate integration of everyday chores and exercise in their lifestyle unveils a critical aspect of their wholesome wellness narrative. Acknowledging the mind-body connection, we explore how harmonious equilibrium contributes to longevity.

Moving forward, we look at spirituality and emotional wellness with traditional beliefs and practices. Contentment and emotional balance speak volumes about a person's overall health, and they might be cardinal factors in Sardinia's astonishing longevity tale.

The sixth chapter takes a turn towards medical insights and healthcare practices, preventive measures, and unique treatments that reside in Sardinia. By merging traditional with modern healthcare, we gain a glimpse of Sardinia's exclusive approach towards health and wellbeing.

Next, we introduce some vibrant centenarians of Sardinia, sharing their life stories and wisdom. Personal perspectives on longevity add invaluable context and authenticity to our quest for understanding heightened lifelines.

By extending our lens beyond Sardinia, we compare global 'Blue Zones', looking at their commonalities and differences. By doing so, we hope to extract generalizable knowledge applicable globally for human longevity.

In the ninth chapter, we dig into practical Sardinian wisdom that can be applied to overall health enhancement. We lay out the groundwork for creating our life's 'Blue Zone.' However, the path to achieving it carries its challenges and considerations, which we must not ignore.

The conclusion comprehensively summarizes the discoveries made throughout our journey. Reflecting upon the entire journey, the implications, and future research directions materialize their long-lasting narrative of longevity into a legacy that the world can incorporate.

This journey promises to be a compelling exploration, interwoven with Sardinian tales and timeless wisdom. While the primary goal is to investigate the rare longevity seen in Sardinian lives, we also strive to charm our readers with the vibrant warmth of Sardinian culture, the tantalizing flavors of their food, and the inspiring richness of their social structure.

Here's hoping that this expedition provides you with as much joy and amazement as it did for us while researching and compiling this treasure of invaluable knowledge. Welcome on board! Let's explore, learn, and grow together, inspired by the gracious lands of Sardinian longevity.

Chapter 1: The Land of Centenarians

The island of Sardinia, nestled in the Mediterranean Sea, lays claim to an intriguing title; it is the 'Land of Centenarians,' boasting one of the highest rates of centenarian and supercentenarian populations globally. With clusters of villages known as the *Blue Zones*, where the frequency of centenarians is significantly higher, Sardinia's longevity puzzle becomes appealing for those pursuing healthy and long living. Amongst the lush hills and pristine beaches, it's not uncommon to meet remarkably vital individuals, having lived for over a hundred years, engaged in work and social activities. Let's dig deeper into Sardinia's geography and its role in shaping the island's demographics. The juxtaposition of rugged mountains and serene coastlines, coupled with a climate that teeters between Mediterranean and continental, fosters a lifestyle that is both active and sedentary, offering a captivating blend of mental peace and physical labor. Then there's a delve into Sardinia's rich history, where invasions, isolation, and agricultural traditions have left indelible marks on the life expectancy of its residents.

The distinct culture further bolsters Sardinia's secret to long life, embodying values and norms that have been passed down through countless generations. This chapter offers a gaze into the land that seems to have unlocked the code to a healthy and prolonged life.

Geography and Demographics

Positioned smack in the middle of the Mediterranean Sea, Sardinia is the second-largest island in this body of water. Its defined geographical boundaries have significantly shaped the island's unique demographic and environmental scenario, aspects of which have proven deeply interwoven with the islanders' remarkable longevity.

The island is predominantly mountainous, with a massif of granite and schist rocks running through the length of the island, dotted with broad plateaus and rugged cliffs plummeting towards the sparkling sea. This challenging, at times even inhospitable, terrain engendered a subsistence-based lifestyle amongst the islanders that revolved around shepherding and small-scale farming.

As for climate, Sardinia enjoys a Mediterranean climate characterized by cool, wet winters and hot, dry summers which directly impacts the local fauna and flora. This untamed Sardinian environment, while challenging for human inhabitants, provides for a diet rich in wild greens, olives, nuts, and berries - all of which contribute critical nutrients to the islanders' diet.

The influence of geography on the demographics of Sardinia is infinitely intertwined. Historically, due to its rough, mountainous terrain, the island was divided into small, remote communities, a tradition that persists to this day.

The majority of Sardinia's centenarians reside in the rural Nuoro province, an area of Sardinia also known as 'barbagia' — a region rich in traditions and folklore. It is estimated that one out of every 250 residents here lives to be a centenarian — a concentration of centenarians which eclipses that of almost every other place in the world.

Shaped by its mountainous topography, Sardinia is not heavily populated, with most residents living in smaller towns and villages. The island's population, which numbers over one million, is fairly evenly distributed - a demographic characteristic that has played a vital role in the perpetuation of traditional lifestyles and practices.

The demographic composition of the island is also unique in comparison to the rest of Italy and the world. Sardinia boasts more male centenarians than virtually any other place on Earth. Typically, globally inclusive, women tend to outlive men. However, in Sardinia, the ratio of centenarian men to women is nearly 1:1, a demographic phenomenon warranting closer analysis.

This unique male-to-female ratio has become a key point of interest for scientists and researchers. Some attribute these higher rates of male longevity to the historical need for physical work such as shepherding and manual farming, work that endowed men with consistent, moderate physical activity throughout their lives. The outdoor nature of these jobs also provided plenty of exposure to sunlight, and thus a frequent supply of Vitamin D.

The isolation of the island has resulted in a gene pool that is more homogenous than most other populations around the world. This homogeny can have significant implications for longevity. Because of a smaller genetic pool, beneficial genes, such as those promoting longevity, have a greater likelihood of being passed down to successive generations.

Social demographics also play a major role in Sardinian longevity. The island's strong sense of community, the proverbial 'everyone knows everyone' phenomena, ensures that villagers look out for one another. There are no 'forgotten' elders in Sardinia. Everyone takes part in the responsibility of caring for older family members or neighbors.

How the island's geographical attributes have influenced its demographic patterns proves revealing in relation to the longevity of its inhabitants. The insularity and ruggedness of the terrain have preserved a unique lifestyle that shields inhabitants from the frenzied pace of modernity. Perhaps, it is this unhurried pace, so deeply linked to the landscape, that contributes in part to the serenity and longevity of its endured inhabitants.

Indeed, it's the combination of both the geography and demographics of Sardinia that gives the region its distinctive character. These factors together influence the local diet, environmental conditions, and social structures, which in turn significantly impact the health and longevity of Sardinians.

So, by unearthing the relationship between Sardinia's specific geographical and demographic situation, we can add one more piece to the jigsaw puzzle of Sardinian longevity.

Historical Background

The story of Sardinia as one of the world's leading Blue Zones begins thousands of years ago. Historically, Sardinia was not always the beacon of health and longevity that it is today. As an island, it has experienced periods of relative isolation and hardship, which unknowingly set the foundations for a culture centered on longevity.

Firstly, Sardinia's geographical location has played a significant role in its history. Situated in the middle of the Mediterranean Sea, the island has served as a crossroad of cultures throughout the millennia. This led to a melting pot of different customs and traditions that have come to define the Sardinian way of life.

Archaeological evidence reveals that Sardinia was inhabited by humans as early as the Paleolithic and Neolithic periods. The Nuragic civilization, which developed in Sardinia around 1800 BC, is proof of the island's ancient heritage. This civilization is still evident today through the thousands of "nuraghe" stone tower-fortresses scattered throughout the island.

Dominated by a multitude of foreign powers over the centuries, Sardinia has historically been an object of conquest due to its strategic location. It fell under the rule of various empires, including the Phoenicians, Romans, Byzantines, Vandals, and later the Spanish and Italians. Each of these cultures left an indelible imprint on the island that remains visible to this day.

For centuries, Sardinians lived as shepherds and farmers, adhering to a traditional lifestyle that largely revolved around the land. Their diet was primarily plant-based, complemented by lean meats from animals they raised and fish caught from the surrounding sea. This pattern of eating, which is the basis of the modern Mediterranean diet, has been linked to health and longevity.

Importantly, these hardy Sardinians faced a challenging environment with limited resources. These hardships became the catalyst for their development of a strong sense of community and family, as cooperation was often necessary for survival. Families and communities came together to share everything they had, and multi-generational households became the norm.

Sardinian society has managed to retain these cultural traditions up to the present day. The close-knit communities and their dedication to mutual aid and hard work have not waned over time. These values have played a pivotal role in the distinctive characteristics that define Sardinia as a Blue Zone.

Social structure also contributes to longevity in Sardinia. Extended family networks provide social and emotional support, which has been proven to significantly impact physical health and longevity. The island's historical emphasis on community support and interdependence directly correlates with the high number of centenarians found within its borders.

The geographical isolation of Sardinia has both shaped and protected its unique societal characteristics. Its relative remoteness has limited the reach of fast food culture and the influence of certain modern convenience technologies, both of which can undermine health and longevity. Historically, this has resulted in limited exposure to lifestyle diseases common in many Western societies.

Over the years, the Sardinian way of life has remained relatively untouched by the rapid pace of modern development that's common on the mainland. This resistance to change, born out of their isolation and self-sufficiency, has inadvertently allowed for the preservation of traditional habits that promote health and longevity.

However, Sardinia's relative obscurity came to an abrupt end in 2000 when scientist Gianni Pes identified the island's northeastern region of Barbagia as a longevity hotspot. Researchers from all around the world began flocking to Sardinia to understand the secrets of its inhabitants' extraordinary longevity.

This attention has led to a surge in interest in the Sardinian lifestyle and diet. Still, the Sardinians remain protective of their culture and traditions. They respect the ways of their ancestors who laid the foundation for their healthy ways of life. This blend of openness to scientific research while still prioritizing and honoring their cultural heritage has kept Sardinia on the map as a fascinating longevity hotspot.

In summary, Sardinia's cultural, geographical, and historical context has crafted a society that values family, community, tradition, and health. These attributes culminate in a populace with an exceptionally high proportion of healthy centenarians. Their experience provides valuable insights into humanity's pursuit of improved health and increased longevity.

Looking back on Sardinia's history, it's clear that the region's unique past has contributed significantly to its present-day status as a Blue Zone. History, it seems, may indeed hold the keys to longevity, with the historical background of Sardinia painting a compelling picture of how external variables can shape a society's health perspective over time.

Cultural Insights

A central aspect of Sardinian society is rooted in its cultural insights, not merely as lofty theories, but as daily life practices that lend to their long-lasting health and longevity. Culture, in this context, is not limited to shared customs or traditions but embodies the community's core ethos to a life lived long and well.

One of the initial remarkable aspects of Sardinian culture is the concept of 'Arai,' a code of behavior that advocates respect, hospitality, humility, and integrity. The Arai encourages individuals to live life with dignity while maintaining respectful relationships with others. These principles form the backbone of Sardinian society and often influence the general approach towards daily routines, interpersonal relationships, and decision-making.

Another cornerstone of Sardinian lifestyle is centered around the notion of family. The structure of the family unit is critical and often composed of multiple generations living under the same roof. This living arrangement promotes intergenerational bonding, leading to a profound sense of respect for elders, their wisdom, and their life experiences. The close-knit family structure also ensures that the elderly are cared for in their later years, enhancing their emotional wellbeing.

In addition to the importance placed on the family, the value of community plays a vital role in Sardinian culture. Villages in Sardinia frequently organize community events, festivals, and local gatherings, fostering a sense of camaraderie and mutual support. This social aspect provides individuals with a sense of purpose and belonging, impacting their overall contentment and longevity positively.

The concept of 'S'imbudu,' meaning, 'reciprocity,' is another cultural insight worth noting. The expectation is that all community members contribute to the shared societal obligations and responsibilities, creating a deeply interwoven web of support and care. This communal sense of responsibility often results in excellent mental well-being, a common factor among the aged Sardinians.

Another integral part of Sardinian culture is the appreciation of nature and physical work. The traditional Sardinian lifestyle has always been centered around pastoral activities and agricultural tasks. Even in today's age of technological advancements, many inhabitants continue to engage in physically demanding tasks as part of their regular routine, contributing significantly to their physical health.

Moreover, the time-honored tradition of storytelling plays a major role in the preservation and distribution of their cultural knowledge. Elders are the revered keepers of history and wisdom and are regularly asked to share stories and experiences, fostering a vibrant oral tradition.

The Sardinians also express their culture through food and drink. Their meals, often shared among family and friends, consist mainly of plant-based ingredients, fresh seafood, and occasionally, meat products, demonstrating an innate respect for the earth's yield. This, coupled with moderate consumption of locally produced wines, paints an idyllic picture of Sardinian dining habits.

Religion, specifically, Catholicism, also weaves itself into the fabric of Sardinian culture. Religious festivals, celebrations, and rituals are commonplace, providing an opportunity for social gatherings and communal bonding, contributing to the people's mental and spiritual wellbeing.

On the same vein, the Sardinian philosophy of life usually embraces tranquility and simplicity. Known as 'Bon'nersu,' it is a joy derived from savoring simple pleasures of life such as enjoying a good meal, relaxing under a tree, or partaking in community festivities.

Sardinians have a remarkable respect for the rhythms of life, governed by the seasons and nature. This understanding and respect for nature's cyclical processes manifest in everything from agriculture to food preparation and daily routines.

'Fortza Paris,' literally meaning 'strength and equality,' is a cultural standard that entails strength of character, fairness in dealings, and tenacity in the face of challenges. It encapsulates the endurance and resilience intrinsic to the Sardinian people, possibly contributing to their long lives.

Finally, an overarching theme in Sardinian culture is the focus on quality of life, as opposed to the relentless pursuit of wealth or prestige. Happiness is often found in daily routines, communal relationships, and the enjoyment of nature, rather than material possessions.

In conclusion, the cultural insights of the Sardinian people provide a compelling view into their long-lived lives. These principles, woven into their daily lives, seem to create conditions conducive to physical health, mental well-being, and overall contentment, leading to a profound sense of wellness and longevity.

While these practices and philosophies may be culturally specific to Sardinia, they carry universal truths about the important role of community, family, respect for nature, physical activity, and social engagement. For those who wish to understand how to live a long, fulfilled life, Sardinia's cultural insights may serve as an inspiring blueprint.

Chapter 2: The Sardinian Diet

As we journey deeper into the heart of Sardinia's exceptional longevity, we turn our attention to a crucial aspect underpinning their health - the diet. Rooted in Mediterranean eating habits, the Sardinian diet presents a flavor-infused canvas of farm-driven, seasonally available produce and seafood. Typical local ingredients like whole grains, legumes, vegetables, fruits, and lean proteins from fish and lamb form the backbone of this diet. The benefit is two-fold; the diet bears a sheer symphony of tastes while simultaneously functioning as a nutritional powerhouse. Olive oil is a staple, providing heart-healthy fats, and moderate wine consumption, particularly the native Cannonau wine rich in antioxidants, adds a unique spin. An eye-catching variety of Sardinian recipes weaves these ingredients together in nourishing combinations and signifies the heightened place of home cooking and slow food tradition in their culture. Sardinians understand that diet doesn't merely refer to what's on one's plate, it represents a lifestyle. Their eating patterns are also complimented by other habits like regular physical activity and strong community ties, contributing to a synergistic effect on longevity. Emphasizing the role of diet in longevity, studies have connected it to lower rates of heart diseases, obesity, cancer, and other chronic illnesses prevalent in western societies. This chapter unveils the beauty of the Sardinian diet, underscoring its nutritious quality which has fostered a populace of centenarians in this blue zone.

Mediterranean Influences

The Mediterranean's vast cultural and geographical span has gifted the world with a rich tapestry of food, lifestyle habits, and attitudes that contribute significantly to longevity. At the heart of it lies Sardinia - an island where these influences are seen, tasted, and lived every day. The Mediterranean influences are intricately woven into Sardinia's fabric, creating a blueprint for remarkable longevity found in its people.

Sardinia is part of the Mediterranean region, sharing climatic, geographical and gastronomic markers with the broader region. The island's isolation has helped to preserve these practices, and it has simultaneously evolved with its unique twist on the Mediterranean habits, contributing to its distinctive longevity.

At the heart of this combined Mediterranean-Sardinian lifestyle is a diet rich in plant-derived foods. Predominantly vegetarian, it espouses whole grains, fresh fruits and vegetables, beans, nuts, and healthy fats sourced mainly from olive oil. The inclusion of fish, thanks to Sardinia's coastal location, along with minimal servings of meat, completes the food cycle.

Root vegetables like chickpeas, lentils, and fava beans are a significant food source. Freshly harvested produce creates a vibrantly colored mosaic on the Sardinian tables - tomatoes, lettuce, zucchinis, aubergines, and several rural herbs. Bread, often homemade, is a staple, as well as pasta. Olive oil serves as the universal dressing, adding subtle flavors and essential fats.

The moderate intake of red wine, particularly Cannonau, a variety typical to the island, is credited with high antioxidant levels that protect against aging. The wine's polyphenols are thought to contribute to reducing heart disease risks, a common cause of mortality elsewhere.

Sardinians observe a simple yet effective food philosophy centered on locally grown, seasonal, and organic items where possible. This concept of 'zero-kilometer' food reduces food mileage and ensures fresher, nutrient-rich food reaches their plates. With less reliance on processed or packaged goods, the diet remains low in bad fats and sugars, thus serving older age brackets well.

Food preparation in Sardinia also resonates with Mediterranean influences. Cooking is more often than not a slow, leisurely process, bringing families together. Fresh ingredients are cooked using traditional methods, retaining most of the nutritional benefits.

Beyond dietary habits, the Mediterranean lifestyle embraces a relaxed pace of life. Emphasis on family bonding, deep social connections, and frequent engagement in communal activities fosters a strong sense of belonging, reducing stress levels and indirectly promoting healthier living.

Mediterranean people also value the concept of 'siesta', a leisurely mid-afternoon rest coinciding with the day's hottest hours. This practice can rejuvenate the body, allowing it to restore energy for the rest of the day and contributing to a balanced lifestyle.

The respect for nature and the earth is another notable Mediterranean trait witnessed in Sardinia. This respect translates into a hardworking demeanor and a close affinity for agriculture, animal herding and outdoor activities, all of which contribute to physical fitness.

Lastly, it is worth noting the tangible sense of contentment that permeates Mediterranean societies, particularly in Sardinia. Achieving happiness isn't associated with materialistic pursuits but rather with leading a fulfilling, balanced life. This emotional wellness contributes to overall health, well-being, and longer life.

Through the ages, Mediterranean communities, including Sardinia, have intuitively followed a way of life that aligns with current scientific understanding of the factors promoting longevity. They have shown us that the secret to a long life may not lie in expensive potions or radical lifestyle changes, but in something as simple as the food we eat, the connections we nurture, and our attitude towards life.

Understanding these influences and incorporating them into one's lifestyle could potentially hold the key to emulation of the longstanding Sardinian success in longevity. However, these should be adapted to personal circumstances and environments to create a relatable and sustainable approach.

In conclusion, the widely admired Sardinian longevity isn't an inexplicable phenomenon but a culmination of various Mediterranean influences. Recognizing and learning from these influences can guide us closer to replicating Sardinia's success and create a blueprint for sustainable, healthier, and longer life.

Local Ingredients and Recipes

The local ingredients and traditional recipes of Sardinia are an essential component of Sardinian longevity. The abundance of vibrant, nutrient-dense, and non-processed agricultural products is deeply connected with the locals' health.

Central to the Sardinian diet is bread (Pane Carasau), made from cultivated grains like barley, wheat, and rye. This bread is made with no preservatives or additives, an example of the simplicity and purity of Sardinian food.

Another staple is the Sardinian pasta known as malloreddus. Made from semolina flour and water, it's often topped with a tomato-based sauce and sprinkled with pecorino cheese. This high fiber, protein-filled meal is tastefully satisfying and nutritionally balanced.

The culinary landscape in Sardinia wouldn't be complete without its distinctive cheeses, like the world-renowned pecorino sardo, made from local sheep's milk. This sharp, tangy delight, is high in protein and calcium and an example of the integral role dairy products play in the Sardinian diet.

Meat isn't the main event in Sardinian cuisine, but when it is consumed, it's high quality, local, and often wild. Roasted pork, in particular, is popular among Sardinians. It is eaten in fair amounts during parties and celebrations, but not on a daily basis. This mindful meat consumption makes it another attribute that contributes to the dietary balance.

Phoenix and blueberries are another critical part of the Sardinian diet. These are bursting with valuable antioxidants that promote health and longevity, contributing to the locals' long lives.

Additionally, legumes like chickpeas and fava beans form part of many traditional Sardinian dishes. They are an excellent source of plant-based protein and fiber, contributing to balanced nutrition.

Fennel, artichokes, tomatoes, eggplants, and zucchinis are just some of the local vegetables that are densely packed with essential nutrients. They're often served fresh, added to stews, or baked into pies.

Fish, primarily bluefin tuna and sardines, is another essential element of the Sardinian diet. It's no surprise, considering the island's location in the Mediterranean Sea. Locals benefit from the omega-3 fatty acids found in these fish, which are known to promote cardiovascular health.

Traditional recipes often incorporate these ingredients, as seen in Sardinian Minestrone, a vegetable and legume soup that has been a staple in Sardinian households for centuries. This hearty, nutrient-dense dish represents the nutritional wisdom of Sardinian cuisine.

Su Porcheddu, roasted suckling pig, is a treat reserved for special occasions and celebrations. This acknowledges the value of moderation in meat consumption.

Seadas is a traditional Sardinian dessert made from cheese-filled semolina dough, fried, and topped with honey. While it's a high-calorie treat, it indicates that no food group is entirely off-limits, including sweets eaten in moderation.

Bottarga di Muggine, fish roe from Mullet often grated over pasta dishes, showcases the locals' ability to use every part of the produce, thus reducing waste and increasing nutritional diversity.

All these ingredients and dishes speak of the Sardinian way of eating - fresh, local, and balanced. There's a deep respect for the land which feeds them, and an understanding that their diet contributes significantly to their remarkable longevity.

In conclusion, the locally sourced, simple, and fresh ingredients coupled with traditional Sardinian recipes offer a rich tapestry of health-boosting, longevity-promoting food. Consuming seasonal, organic, and minimally processed dishes keeps the Sardinians vibrant, energetic, and mentally sharp well into their later years. Through their diet, we see their connection to the earth, their love for good food, and their commitment to a high-quality life.

The Role of Diet in Longevity

Diet unquestionably plays a pivotal role in longevity, as it significantly influences our overall physical health, cognitive ability, and emotional vitality. A healthful, balanced diet particularly lays the groundwork for optimal body function and longevity. In the Sardinian context, their diet is one form of the Mediterranean diet, which is universally recognized for its essential contributions to health and well-being.

Sardinians consume a predominantly plant-based diet abundant in whole grains, fruits, and vegetables. This implies a high intake of dietary fiber and antioxidants, which contribute to overall health by reducing the risk of chronic diseases. Such an eating plan also includes an ample amount of legumes, which act as a valuable source of protein and also help regulate blood sugar levels.

The hallmark of the Sardinian diet is longevity bread, known locally as 'pane carasau.' It's a type of flatbread made from whole grains and has fewer calories compared to other bread varieties. With its high fiber content, this bread aids digestion and keeps one satiated for longer periods, thereby preventing overeating, a leading factor contributing to obesity and other health issues.

Another essential element in the Sardinian diet is goat's milk and pecorino cheese made from it. Goat's milk is rich in omega-3 fatty acids and antioxidants, which can slow down aging, counter inflammation, and protect against heart disease. Additionally, pecorino cheese derived from grass-fed sheep milk in Sardinia has high levels of CLA (Conjugated Linoleic Acid), a fatty acid known to possess various health benefits, including enhancing immune function and preventing certain types of cancer.

The Sardinians have a habitual intake of red wine, especially Cannonau wine, known for its high polyphenol content that has heart-friendly properties. Consuming moderate amounts of this wine can have a dual effect - firstly, it's antioxidant-rich nature aids in fighting harmful inflammation in the body. Secondly, the ritual of wine consumption enhances social engagement and de-stresses, which also contribute to longevity.

Olive oil rounds up the diet in the Sardinian longevity equation. It's a powerhouse of monounsaturated fats, more specifically oleic acid, which has been linked to reduced heart disease risk. Moreover, extra virgin olive oil is rich in antioxidants that fight inflammation and help protect LDL (bad) cholesterol from oxidation.

While the constituents of the diet play a critical role, it is equally important to consider the Sardinian food philosophy. Sardinians practice mindful eating, where they take time to appreciate and savor their food, often in the company of friends and family. This not only enhances digestion but also encourages social connections, which are an integral part of longevity.

Portion control is another aspect of eating in Sardinia that impacts longevity. Sardinians often consume small plates of food, avoiding large meals, especially in the late evening. This practice aids digestion and helps maintain a healthy body weight.

Additionally, Sardinians source most of their food locally, ensuring that they consume the freshest and most-nutritious food possible. The use of home-grown produces and locally raised animals means that their diet is devoid of processed foods, which are known accelerators of aging.

However, it's important not to interpret the Sardinian diet as a 'magic bullet' for longevity. While it does significantly contribute to achieving it, their diet does not exist in isolation from their other lifestyle factors. Exercise, social interaction, and healthy emotional wellbeing work synergistically with diet to promote lifespan-extending benefits.

From a wider perspective, the impact of diet on longevity isn't solely limited to the types of foods one consumes. It also involves how and when one eats, along with the overarching philosophy one holds towards nutrition and health. It's about balance and enjoying what you eat while still feeding your body the nutrients it needs for optimal health.

In a nutshell, the Sardinian diet demonstrates that eating isn't just about fueling our bodies but also connecting with our communities, respecting nature's bounty, and savoring its flavors. Their diet doesn't provide a prescriptive template to follow but rather offers inspiring principles for healthful eating that can contribute to longevity wherever one resides.

Longevity is a holistic outcome of multiple lifestyle factors working in harmony. The Sardinian approach to diet admirably illustrates how enjoyable and sociable eating habits, combined with balanced and nutritious food choices, align perfectly with overall longevity. To live a long and vibrant life, one should draw lessons from the Sardinian dietary practices, fit them into their culture and personal preferences and adapt over time for sustained benefits.

Chapter 3: Family and Social Ties

As we delve into the deeper layers of Sardinia's longevity phenomenon, we find that the importance of robust social bonds cannot be overstated. The Sardinian culture nurtures both familial relationships and communal ties, forming a woven tapestry of social support and connection. The value they place on family extends beyond nuclear units, often encompassing extended relatives and sometimes the entire village. Interactions and mutual support among different generations contribute to a sense of belonging and emotional security, reinforcing the relevance of **family structures** in this narrative. Simultaneously, their potent communal spirit fosters a sense of social responsibility and solidarity, further strengthening the ties that bind the community together. Residents engage in daily social rituals and community activities, which not only serve to reinforce their cultural identity but also provide cognitive stimulation and emotional well-being, demonstrating the significance of **social engagement** for mental health. Hence, these facets of Sardinian society seem to play an integral role in the longevity of their population, underscoring an often overlooked aspect of healthy and prolonged life - the power of familial and social ties.

The Importance of Community

Now more than ever, we're beginning to appreciate the immense value of community in fostering connections and laying the foundation for a fulfilling life. This is especially true in areas known as 'Blue Zones,' geographic locations celebrated for their high concentration of centenarians. Here we'll delve into the role that community plays in longevity, particularly focusing on Sardinia, a global blue zone.

In Sardinia, often referred to as the 'Land of Centenarians,' the adage 'it takes a village to raise a child' takes on a deeper meaning. The cohesion, mutual support, and deep connections fostered within communities are integral to Sardinian life. It's not just about individual longevity - the vitality of the entire community is a priority. Community is viewed as the beating heart, the life fuel that allows individuals to weather hardships, celebrate victories, and grow old together.

Children are nurtured by an entire community, continually exposed to the wisdom and experiences of the older generation. This intergenerational integration shapes mindsets, behaviors, and attitudes, maintaining a cultural continuum that prioritizes family, community, and a slower pace of life.

Active participation within the community is another hallmark of Sardinian life. Whether through religious customs, local festivals, or the simple act of daily socializing, there's a sense of being involved and invested in the life of the community that deepens relationships, diminishes loneliness, and promotes a supportive, communal spirit.

However, the importance of community isn't limited solely to social aspects. Communities also provide a context for shared responsibilities and duties that often involve physical activity. Tasks such as tending to local gardens, livestock, vineyards, and other such activity bind the community members together while keeping them physically active—a key factor to longevity.

This notion of community interconnectedness extends to meal times as well. Sardinian meals are usually communal experiences shared with family or friends—not solitary endeavors endured in front of a screen. The socializing during meals slows the eating process, encouraging a more mindfully engaged and satisfied approach towards food.

Communities in Sardinia also demonstrate an elegant balance between tradition and progress. While they embrace change and the opportunities it brings, they're also deeply rooted in historic traditions, passing down carefully preserved cultural practices from generation to generation.

The value of tradition in Sardinian communities is particularly evident in their approach to local produce and recipes, using seasonal and organic ingredients—an essential element to their famed Mediterranean diet. Food is not just nourishment; it embodies tradition, pride of place, and family heritage.

What's also stunning about the Sardinian community spirit is its profound empathy. The Sardinians refer to it as 's'aja,' a unique blend of empathy, patience, tolerance, and respect. This behavior is taught early in life and perpetuated through time, echoing the idea of shared hardships and joys.

Community importance for mental health cannot be understated. In Sardinia, there's a lower incidence of depression, anxiety, and stress-related ailments compared to other regions. This can be linked back to the support systems in place at the community level, providing a cushion against mental health issues and helping individuals navigate life's challenges more effectively.

While it isn't new information that community is essential for mental wellbeing, the Sardinian example presents an enlightening perspective. Community isn't just a loosely connected group of individuals living in proximity. It's a deeply rooted network of relationships that preserve traditions, values, and connection—a latticework of lives interwoven through shared experiences, cultures, food, and age-old wisdom.

The Sardinians' strong emphasis on community illuminates a fundamental, often neglected aspect of health and wellbeing: social connections are over as pivotal as dietary habits and physical activities in the pursuit of longevity. For Sardinians, community isn't a convenience; it's a necessity, a lifeblood flowing through the veins of the entire society.

In essence, the small communities of Sardinia unveil a quantum leap understanding of longevity. Their collective wisdom affirms that while diet, physical activity, and medical care are significant elements in the longevity blueprint, they're ultimately part of a larger tapestry that is held together and infused with richness by the bonds of community.

So, as we delve deeper into Sardinia's secret to longevity, don't mistake it as just a series of health tips and lifestyle adjustments. It's a testament to how living connected with others, grounded in a strong community spirit, can shape our lives, influence our wellbeing, and indeed make us richer —in body, mind, and soul.

Family Structures and Relationships

In Sardinia, the fabric of family life is tightly woven and persists through generations. Family structures and relationships are a key factor in maintaining the island's community identity and individual health. This may be one of their well-kept secrets to longevity.

At the heart of Sardinian home life, respect for the elderly is intrinsic. Unlike in many Western societies, where elderly people are often placed in retirement homes, Sardinia has a longstanding tradition of multigenerational living. Children, parents, and grandparents often share the same house, creating a nurturing and supportive environment for all family members.

This model of family living offers immediate benefits to both the young and old. The elderly get to revel in the youthfulness and vigor of the younger family members. Meanwhile, children are enriched by the wisdom and life experience of their grandparents. This exchange cultivates strong familial bonds and a robust social safety net.

The Sardinian culture has a unique concept known as "teachings of ancestors." Intergenerational living enables the effortless transfer of the 'teachings of ancestors' from the older generation to the younger ones - a process that creates cultural cohesion and stability.

Family structures also shape the meal times in Sardinia. Families regularly gather around the table to enjoy meals together. The dining table is a central meeting place where family members can bond, exchange stories, and cultivate strong relationships.

On the flip side, this strong family-oriented culture does not limit individual agency or independence. Indeed, Sardinians tend to enjoy high levels of autonomy, with individual roles respected and responsibilities clearly defined within the familial matrix. This balance of interdependence and autonomy might contribute to a sense of life satisfaction and consequently longer life.

Additionally, the nature of familial ties in Sardinia indicates an unwavering commitment to kinship. This commitment is often evidenced by the readiness of family members to provide assistance, whether it be financial help or child care, whenever necessary. This mutual support can mitigate the impact of adverse life events and promote resilience and well-being.

Furthermore, the role of gender cannot be ignored when discussing Sardinian family structures and relationships. The traditionally patriarchal society has seen substantial shifts over the years, moving towards gender balance and equality. This has resulted in men and women sharing the caregiving and financial responsibilities that come with family life.

Yet, in Sardinia, women often remain the caregivers in the family and the main agents of emotional support. They play an essential role in maintaining family relationships and fostering a strong sense of kinship. Therefore, women's contribution to family life could be viewed as another pillar supporting Sardinian longevity.

On the whole, Sardinian family systems place a strong emphasis on cooperation and mutual support. Rather than being isolated units, families in Sardinia are interconnected threads in a larger community tapestry, fostering a sense of belonging and emotional security among all members.

This isn't just about pure sentimentality, though. Research has shown that strong familial bonds can have tangible health benefits, including lower stress levels, better mental health, and increased longevity. Sardinians seem to understand this intuitively and have allowed these principles to guide their family relationships.

In summary, the tightly-knit family structures and robust kinship ties present in Sardinian society create a sense of security, continuity, and affection, which shape both individual and collective well-being. These qualities seem to have a profound influence on longevity and life satisfaction among the population.

The Sardinian model of familial bonds offers a compelling contrast to the often individualistic tendencies of the modern Western world. It serves as a reminder that, as humans, we're inherently social creatures who thrive in nurturing, supportive communities.

The effect of these familial and relational factors on longevity in Sardinia underscores the importance of holistic wellbeing. It appears that it's not just diet, exercise, or healthcare that matter - there's a strong case for the idea that close familial bonds, respect for the elderly, and nurturing relationships can all contribute significantly to a long and healthy life.

Despite cultural and societal differences, the essence of the Sardinian family structure - the love, support, mutual respect, and sense of belonging - can be universal. The Sardinians offer a path that, if adopted wherever applicable, could enrich lives, strengthen family bonds, and promote psychological health, thereby positively impacting overall longevity.

Social Engagement and Mental Health

As we delve deeper into the constituents of the unique Sardinian way of life that contributes to their exceptional longevity, one can't help but notice the remarkable degree of social integration prevalent within these communities. This integrative social lifestyle seems to play a crucial part in the overall mental health of the inhabitants and warrants further exploration.

To begin, let us take a closer look at how social engagement is woven into the fabric of daily life in Sardinia. Unlike the often isolated existence many individuals in western societies experience, Sardinians tend to live in tight-knit communities where social interaction is a fundamental part of day-to-day life. From helping each other in farming tasks to the traditional evening passeggiata, also known as an evening stroll, where villagers walk and chat with each other, social engagement is omnipresent.

The significant aspect about these interactions is that it's not just about superficial niceties but shared experiences and real connections. There's a sense of camaraderie and mutual respect that binds these communities together. It is this sense of belonging that fosters a positive mindset, contributing to overall mental well-being.

This interconnectedness extends beyond immediate family and friends to include the entire community. It is common for village residents to know each other personally, with opportunities for socializing embedded in their daily routines. As such, solitude is scarce, and uninvolvement is unlikely, contributing to a reduced risk of loneliness and mental health issues.

Social engagement in Sardinia is not just about connections, but support systems too. When someone faces a challenge or suffers a loss, the community bands together to provide support. This practice further enhances an individual's resilience to stress and helps maintain mental equanimity.

The mental health benefits of such social engagement are plentiful. The constant interaction and emotional support can lessen instances of anxiety, depression, and stress. Moreover, the diverse conversations and experiences fostered by this social climate can help keep the mind agile and healthy even as individuals age, guarding against cognitive decline and boosting mental energy.

Interestingly, the social engagement that thrives in Sardinia cuts across all age groups, sustaining the mental well-being of both young and old residents. Teenagers, adults, and centenarians alike participate in community affairs, often learning from one another. This intergenerational bonding promotes empathy, understanding, and respect for elders and brings balance and perspective to the younger generation.

Equally essential is the role of the elderly in these social dynamics. Sardinians greatly respect and venerate the aged, who are frequently consulted for advice and valued for the wisdom and experience they bring to the community. Far from being cast aside or marginalized, the elderly remain influential members of the society: vibrant, engaged, and cognitively active.

This approach contrasts sharply with the typical Western attitude, where often, aging is perceived as a drawback and older individuals are isolated. In Sardinia, age is seen as a testament to a life well-lived, accruing wisdom, and contributing positively to society. The recognition and inclusion of the elderly in social activities further contribute to their mental well-being and overall sense of satisfaction.

Now, what can we learn from the Sardinian approach to social engagement? For starters, the importance of cultivating and maintaining connections cannot be overstressed. Irrespective of the size and location of your community, fostering a sense of cohesion and mutual support goes a long way in promoting positive mental health.

Furthermore, taking part in shared community activities, and involving all age groups, from kids to the elderly, can enhance the richness of these connections. Not only does it promote understanding across generations, but it also fosters a diverse and nourishing social landscape.

Finally, the value of viewing aging as an asset rather than a liability underscores the importance of respecting and including the elderly in the social matrix. Treating them as vital elements of the community and drawing on their wisdom and experience isn't just beneficial for their mental health but can enrich society as a whole.

In conclusion, Sardinian's unique approach to social engagement offers invaluable lessons for enhancing mental health. It underlines the power of community, the importance of inclusive social structures, the countering of isolation, and the celebration of age, all of which significantly contribute to mental well-being.

While the structural mechanisms that support these social norms aren't easily transferrable, we can certainly aspire to imbibe these principles in our personal lives and communities. Recognizing the profound connection between social engagement and mental health is a critical step on the journey to healthier, longer lives.

Chapter 4: Active Living and Physical Well-being

In Chapter 3, we explored the role of social connections and family ties in promoting longevity. As we delve into Chapter 4, the focus shifts to the importance of an active lifestyle and overall physical well-being. The day-to-day routines of the Sardinians promote constant movement, with activities ranging from pastoral duties, to gardening, to house chores, which are integral to their living standards. These tasks might seem mundane, but they actually nourish the Sardinian's resilience and contribute to their physical strength well into old age. Besides daily tasks, formal exercises such as walking and hiking are also a fundamental part of life in this Mediterranean island, not only strengthening muscles but also connecting them to their picturesque surroundings. The exploration of such active living is not merely a study of physical endurance or strength, but also the connection between the body and mind. The Sardinian's physical activities are often intertwined with social interactions and connections to nature, fostering a sense of purpose, enhancing mental health, and nurturing a positive attitude towards aging. This close connection, between daily practices, physical wellness and mental health, could be a key element in unlocking why the people of Sardinia have such an impressive longevity record.

Daily Routines and Work

Life in the blue zones, specifically in Sardinia, significantly differs from the rushed, stress-filled lives commonly found in the urbanized parts of the globe. Sardinians live deeply connected with the land and the seasons, and this bond is prominent in their daily routines and working life. These routines have a strong impact on their overall health and longevity.

Many Sardinians work in professions that may be considered physically challenging. Farmers, shepherds, and fishermen make up a large chunk of the working population. This kind of labor necessitates regular movement and physical activity, ensuring that people remain active throughout their lives. As opposed to sedentary jobs, these naturally active professions promote a healthier lifestyle by keeping people physically engaged, helping them maintain a healthy weight, and reducing the risk of chronic diseases.

Another critical aspect of the Sardinians' daily routine is their adherence to a natural rhythm of life. This concept of living might be best encompassed by the Sardinian phrase "A su Sardu no bi at nessi ischida," which translates to "The Sards do not let themselves be rushed." In this culture, there's an integrated practice of taking time to rest and recharge, often with an afternoon 'siesta' or nap. This accommodates for needed rest, reducing instances of chronic fatigue and stress.

Mealtimes in Sardinia are not just occasions for nourishment, but also for socializing, relaxing, and enjoying life. These meals are usually prolonged affairs, savored with family members or friends. Unlike the rushed meals that many of us are used to, Sardinians take the time to truly appreciate their food and the company they share it with. This has been shown to aid digestion and promote a feeling of satisfaction and contentment, which in turn reduces overeating and helps maintain a healthy weight.

Sardinians also integrate regular walks into their routine, whether these be for daily commuting to their fields or just a stroll through the village. Walking has been proven to have numerous health benefits, including improving cardiovascular health, strengthening bones, losing weight, and boosting mental well-being. They also frequently participate in communal activities that bolster physical health, such as local festivals which often revolve around dancing.

An important feature of Sardinian work-life is "passione"— nothing short of a passion for their work. Sardinians not only work to make a living but also draw a deep sense of purpose and satisfaction from their labor. This attachment to work gives them a sense of identity, fosters resilience, and aids their physical and mental well-being.

Among Sardinians, the divide between work and non-work hours is often blurred. Work in this context does not feel like a burden or something to get done with. Instead, it's thought of as an integral part of life, something that's done at a natural pace and enjoyed heartily.

Many of their daily pursuits involve interaction with nature. Whether it's tending to animal herds, cultivating crops, or gathering herbs for cooking, these activities keep Sardinians grounded and provide an echo back to their ancestral lifestyle. They use traditional tools in their work, again promoting physical activity and reducing reliance on machinery.

Intergenerational interaction is another widespread facet of Sardinian daily life. It's common to find multiple generations living under one roof or in close proximity. Older generations often contribute to the family's income by indulging in tasks suitable for their age, like tending to the garden, cooking, or helping with childcare. This allows them to remain active, valued, and engaged in their community.

Furthermore, evenings in Sardinia are often spent communally, where villagers gather in local bars or squares to chat, play games, and enjoy each other's company. Such social interactions act as stress-relievers and contribute to their overall sense of happiness and life satisfaction.

The routines followed by the Sardinians provide incredible insights into the views and approaches towards daily activities and work. As such, attempting to emulate these elements in our lives could prove beneficial. Many of us have jobs that entail long hours of sitting, and we are disconnected from nature, community, and even family. We could certainly learn a lot from the Sardinian approach to daily routines and work.

Ultimately, it's clear that the Sardinians' daily routines work harmoniously, enhancing their well-being in a holistically sustainable way. Their routines keep them physically active, mentally engaged, socially connected, and emotionally content, contributing significantly to their globally-renowned longevity.

In the realm of the Sardinian lifestyle, work is not separate from life; rather, it is seamlessly woven into the fabric of everyday. This interplay between work, rest, social interaction, and connection with nature found in the daily routines of Sardinians, appears to be an essential component of achieving not just longevity, but a joyful and fulfilling life.

We would do well to heed these principles as we navigate the demands of our modern lives. Adopting practices such as spending more time outdoors, ensuring regular physical activity, slowing down our pace, making time for community interaction, and eating together can have profound and positive impacts on our health and longevity.

Physical Activities and Exercise

The inhabitants of Sardinia's Blue Zones stand testimony to the fact that physical activity is crucial to a long, healthy life. It's not about gym memberships, high-intensity workouts, or sports prowess, but about integrating regular, moderate activity into daily life. In the following sections, we'll go deeper into the role of physical activities and exercise in the daily lives of Sardinians.

Sardinians typically lead active lives, with the physical nature of their daily routines acting as a built-in fitness routine. From a young age, they are often involved in physically demanding tasks, particularly those located in rural areas where farming is carried out. This agricultural work forms the backbone of their exercise and keep them active and fit. There's something to be said about the health benefits of staying close to the Earth and leading a life that's intertwined with nature's rhythm.

The Sardinian lifestyle doesn't incorporate exercise as a separate, dedicated part of life. Instead, the general way of life has a natural cadence of physical activity to it. Daily commute in this mountainous region usually involves walking or riding up steep slopes, and houses often don't have modern conveniences, meaning more physical work for everyone. Every day is an opportunity to get the heart rate up, burn calories, and flex muscles without intentionally hitting the gym.

The longevity seen in Sardinia shows that long-term low-intensity exercise like walking or tending to the fields is more beneficial than short-term high-intensity workouts. This is primarily because it doesn't put undue stress on the body, thereby reducing the likelihood of cardiovascular incidents and injuries. Such sustained activity also improves endurance and sturdiness which is handy as one ages.

Another significant factor is the physical regimentation of Sardinian occupations. Generations of Sardinian men have been shepherds, spending their days walking across fields and hills in what is essentially a form of mobile meditation. Walking or consistent movement can have a significant impact on both physical and mental health, leading to improved cardiovascular health, lower blood pressure, increased insulin sensitivity, and improved mood.

Apart from the physical exertion involved in work, Sardinians also engage in traditional games and dances. These are not only fun but also act as great communal activities that get everyone moving, regardless of their age. Traditional dance, in particular, combines the benefits of exercise, balance, mobility, coordination, and a social element that's so crucial to longevity.

Maintaining functionality and mobility in the later years is an essential part of good health and personal freedom. Sardinian centenarians typically have a high degree of mobility, sustaining the ability to carry out daily activities and engage with their community. This can be traced back to their consistent lifelong physical activity.

Furthermore, it's vital to note how attitudes towards physical activity contribute to the Sardinian way of life. Exercise isn't seen as a chore, nor is it pursued in the name of vanity. It's merely a natural part of their lifestyle, integrated seamlessly into their lives, which significantly adds to its sustainability.

One can't discuss Sardinian physical activity without mentioning the close ties to nature. Going for hikes in the beautiful Sardinian landscape, swimming in the clear waters surrounding the island or spending time in gardens and fields instill a sense of peace, well-being, and an intuitive understanding of natural rhythms. Regular exposure to sunlight also provides the essential Vitamin D which improves bone health, immunity, and mood regulation.

Aspects of the Sardinian diet also lend themselves to a more active lifestyle. The Mediterranean diet, lower in processed sugars and unhealthy fats, gives the energy required to remain active throughout the day. It ensures that people are less likely to suffer from debilitating conditions that could limit their mobility or general fitness.

Additionally, there's an interesting reciprocal relationship between physical activity and rest. Sardinians understand the importance of balance, valuing leisure, and idle time as much as they do work and physical exertion. This well-rounded approach to life impacts overall wellness, acknowledging that the body and mind both need a certain amount of rest to function optimally.

All of this analysis leads to an important conclusion. People shouldn't force themselves into rigorous, high-intensity workout regimes that they don't enjoy. Instead, like the Sardinians, they should focus on making physical activity a part of their daily activities and hobbies that they love and can sustain over the long term.

As we move on to understanding the connection between body and mind in the next section, keep in mind the importance of activity in promoting longevity. In longevity hotspots like Sardinia, high levels of physical activity are not a lifestyle choice, but a fundamental pillar of life itself.

Let us learn from Sardinia and weave physical activity into our life-tapestry, finding joy, purpose, and health through our actions. Like the Sardinians, we can age with grace, vitality, and strength, fostering both our bodies and the bonds that tie us to our community, our work, and our planet.

Connection between Body and Mind

As we continue our exploration of Sardinian lifestyle and its connection with longevity, we arrive at a pivotal concept - the profound link between body and mind. Through meticulous observation and analysis, scientists have come to appreciate the intimate relationship between our physical and mental well-being. Although this connection may appear straightforward, it requires a deeper understanding to grasp its significance fully.

The people in blue zones, notably Sardinia, appear to have deciphered this intriguing puzzle. They intuitively understand that a holistic approach to health, encompassing both mental and physical wellness is the key to an enriched, prolonged life. The integration of mind and body wellness is palpable in their daily activities, interactions, and overall lifestyle.

Think about the relaxed pace at which life is lived in Sardinia. This unhurried lifestyle aids in stress reduction, promoting a state of calm that benefits both the mind and the body. Stress, as we know, can manifest physically as ailments like heart disease and hypertension. By maintaining a tranquil mind-state, Sardinians actively mitigate such health risks.

The integration of physical activities into their daily lives is another powerful conduit for body-mind wellness. The work of local shepherds, for instance, requires a considerable deal of physical labor. This regular exercise serves to keep them physically fit well into old age while also fostering a positive mental state.

But beyond just habitual exercise, there's a powerful element of mindfulness tagged to it. Whether tending to their gardens or hand-picking olives, Sardinians perform these tasks with heightened awareness. This conscious engagement with their environment and actions is akin to a meditation practice, reinforcing their mind-body connection.

Nurturing social bonds is another facet where the connection between body and mind is visible. Close-knit family structures, active community participation, and regular social engagement are signature traits of blue zones. These networks provide emotional support, alleviate the burden of stress, and catalyze positive mental health, which in turn, impacts physical health positively.

Interestingly, Sardinians also use leisure as a catalyst for mind-body wellness. Their celebration of life through music, dance, food, and communal gatherings are not just social entertainment but avenues for physical activity and mental relaxation. In a world preoccupied with clinical fitness regimes and mental health therapies, such simple yet powerful modes of wellness are worth admiring.

Sardinians have also harnessed nature to maintain the delicate balance between their body and mind. They believe that spending time in nature – walking through hillside paths, tending to their livestock, or cultivating their vegetation – provides not only physical benefits but also mental relaxation and anti-stress effects.

Even on the dietary front, the balanced Mediterranean diet of whole foods, fresh fruits, and vegetables not only nourishes the physical body, but also supports positive mental health. From an outsider's perspective, they're not just feeding their bodies; they're feeding their minds too.

The traditional Sardinian lifestyle does not discriminate between body and mind. They inherently perceive and respect the interplay between both. The older generation pass on this knowledge to younger generations, not as explicit lessons, but as a lifestyle for them to experience and learn.

From a scientific perspective, emerging research in psychoneuroimmunology supports these observations. This interdisciplinary field studies the complex interactions between the nervous system and the immune system, providing evidence for a connection between our mind-states (thoughts, emotions, stress levels) and physical health. These findings validate many of the time-honored mind-body practices observed in blue zones.

In conclusion, the mind-body connection exemplified by the Sardinian lifestyle reflects a profound truth: our health is not merely the absence of disease but a state of complete physical, mental, and social well-being. Numerous scientific studies back this stance, further bolstering the blue zone ethos.

Realizing this connection not only places humanity at the forefront of a revolution in healthcare but also recaptures the essence of being human. As we progress through the book, keep this integrative perspective in mind as we delve deeper into the specifics of mind-body health in the blue zones.

Understanding and adopting this integral mind-body philosophy from the blue zones, such as Sardinia, can be a transformative step toward enhancing our health and longevity. It's a roadmap, guiding us to the understanding that to live long, we must first recognize and respect the symbiotic relationship between our minds and bodies.

Chapter 5: Spiritual and Emotional Wellness

If we shift our gaze inward, we'll find that the Sardinians also possess robust spiritual and emotional wellness, which contributes to their longevity. Traditional beliefs and practices, deeply rooted in respect for nature and the divine, equip them with an unshaken sense of purpose and identity. Through daily prayers, heartfelt songs, and community gatherings, they achieve an intimate connection with the spiritual realm, bringing peace and harmony to their lives. Furthermore, the Sardinians practice mindfulness, effortlessly embedding it into their daily routines. This enables them to savor each moment and derive contentment from the simplest joys. Lastly, this community recognizes the importance of emotional balance for overall health. Managing stress effectively, expressing emotions openly, and building strong social connections are considered key to emotional well-being. Whether it's a bustling Sunday family lunch or an evening chat under the stars with neighbors, there is always laughter, abundant love, and a sense of belonging that nurtures their emotional health.

Traditional Beliefs and Practices

As we delve into the spiritual and emotional wellness of Sardinians, we come across the intriguing role that their traditional beliefs and practices play in their longevity. Rooted deep in their culture, the unique beliefs in Sardinian society have shaped the way inhabitants approach life and their health.

First on the list is the ancient and widespread belief in the 'evil eye.' It's a belief that negative energy from envious persons could result in physical illness or misfortune. To prevent this, many Sardinians - old and young - wear amulets or perform rituals for protection. This practice isn't limited to superstition as it can lead to a reduction in stress levels and bolster a positive outlook, both advantageous for longevity.

Additionally, Sardinia is rich in a myriad of folk beliefs and customs. These practices, handed down over centuries, carry deep meanings connected to nature, family, and the community. Observing taboos, participating in frequent communal feasts, and honoring rituals associated with key life events - birth, weddings, and funerals, all provide a sense of connectedness and mutual support among community members.

Ironically, the key to longevity might be found in funerary traditions. Sardinians have a profound, respectful relationship with death. It's an event marked with elaborate, extended communal rituals, honoring the life lived and facilitating the bereavement process. Understanding death as a natural part of life can eliminate much of the associated fear and anxiety, contributing to emotional balance.

Moreover, the indigenous Sardinian language, 'Nugoresu', contains wisdom about good living and wellbeing which has been passed from generation to generation. Inherent in the language are beliefs and concepts about respect for nature, the value of hard work, and the importance of community. These may help explain the longevity of the Sardinian people.

A high respect for elders is also deeply integrated into their culture. The age-old adage of "respect your elders" is not just a simple phrase but a way of life in Sardinia. The elderly aren't seen as burdens but as essential family members who carry years of wisdom.

Sardinians also believe in 'familismo,' an ideology that heavily emphasizes an individual's obligations and commitment to the family unit. From early on, Sardinians are taught to value their family above all else, including their own individual wants and needs. This belief fosters strong family bonds, providing emotional support and reducing stress, which undeniably contributes to healthier, longer lives.

Perhaps one of the most fascinating traditional practices in Sardinian culture is the art of storytelling. Regarded as an essential trait, the ability to tell a good story is perceived as a sign of wisdom and intelligence. Storytelling sessions promote shared experiences, knowledge transfer, and a strong sense of community among locals, strengthening social bonds and improving mental health.

The practice of gratitude is another significant aspect of the Sardinian lifestyle. They regularly express thanks for what they have, which cultivates a sense of fulfillment, happiness, and contentment. From a scientific perspective, this positive spirit boosts the immune system which contributes to longer lifespans.

Furthermore, Sardinia's religious customs are deeply rooted in Roman Catholicism, with strong blending of ancient traditions. Many Sardinians, particularly the elderly, express a strong faith in God. Pilgrimages to holy sites, donating to the church, and praying regularly are common practices. There is a widespread belief in miracles and divine intervention, which can lead to feelings of hope and optimism - certainly beneficial for longevity.

No discussion about traditional practices would be complete without addressing the customary diet and gardening practices, both of which have been detailed in earlier chapters. From harvesting their own produce, to the communal preparation and enjoyment of meals, Sardinians have preserved a healthful and sustainable way of living that bolsters their longevity.

Lastly, the practice of honoring daily work routines reinforces the value of industriousness in the Sardinian culture. Whether it be tending to the crops, sewing, or grinding wheat, traditional occupations in Sardinia involve physical labor. All these practices enhance physical fitness and keep the mind active, contributing to overall health and wellbeing.

To understand the Sardinian secrets to longevity, it's clear we need to assess their strong cultural beliefs and traditional practices that hold emotional wellness at their core. They form an intricate web, ushering in a collective sense of belonging, fulfillment, and peace of mind. The physical health benefits are but a fortunate side-effect of their emotionally satisfying lifestyle.

In the next section, we take a different angle on Sardinian longevity and delve into the realm of mindfulness and contentment while further exploring the impact of emotional balance on health.

Mindfulness and Contentment

The tranquility of Sardinia's surroundings breeds a disposition of mindfulness and contentment among the inhabitants, a mental state that doubtlessly contributes to their remarkable longevity.

Essentially, mindfulness is the art of being fully engaged in the here and now. It's not so much an act or a state that one achieves, but more of a journey or way of living. In Sardinian culture, mindfulness means investing wholeheartedly in the task at hand—be it a conversation with a family member, labour in the fields, or the simple act of enjoying a meal.

Mindfulness expert Dr. Jon Kabat-Zinn describes it as "paying attention in a particular way, on purpose, in the present moment, and non-judgmentally". This perfectly captures the essence of Sardinian living. Absence of hurry, presence of mind, and a deep engagement with the present moment is a signature trait of the island's community.

This deeply entrenched mindfulness perhaps has its roots in the island's predominant occupation of farming and herding, both activities requiring a meditative labor of love and patience. The island's raw, untouched landscape also creates a sense of awe and wonder that fosters mindfulness.

Moving onto contentment, it is as much an inherent part of the mental makeup of Sardinians as mindfulness. Contentment signifies understanding and appreciating the value of what one has, rather than continuously longing for more. In Sardinia, there is a common phrase "Avere tutto il necessario" which means "Having everything necessary". This subtly reflects their peaceful acceptance of life as it is, content with their day-to-day existence without the constant desire for more.

Sardinians indulge in simple pleasures that are often overlooked in the hustle and bustle of modern life, such as the joy of a shared meal, the beauty of their scenic surroundings, or the soothing rhythm of the sea. Their contentment is not one of complacency or stagnation, but one borne out of a deep appreciation for life and the natural world.

Mindfulness and contentment help create emotional balance, reducing stress and amplifying happiness. This positive relationship with the mind certainly optimizes mental health directly and indirectly affects physical health, fuelling longevity.

Several studies have linked mindfulness practices to decreased levels of stress and anxiety, improved cognition, enhanced emotional regulation, and overall wellbeing. As we have delineated earlier in the role of mindfulness in Sardinian life, these potential health benefits provide strong evidence of its contributory role in the impressive longevity of its inhabitants.

Research also shows a strong correlation between contentment and prolonged lifespan. It is seen that people who remain satisfied with their lives tend to live healthier and longer lives, as contentment can reduce stress and its lethal effects on the body.

Following the Sardinian way, one can cultivate these traits through daily activities. Mindful breathing, concentration, and a conscious effort to savor the present moment are some starting points for mindfulness practice. To foster contentment, it can be helpful to regularly practice gratitude, prioritize relationships, find joy in simplicity, and adapt a positive attitude towards change.

In mitigating the adverse effects of tension and worry, mindfulness and contentness may be the soul's antidote to the perpetuations of the modern world. While we are entangled in the web of external achievements, we can learn from the Sardinians and strive for internal success.

It is therefore important to understand that mindfulness and contentment are not mere buzzwords or quickly achieved states of being, but are rather a way of life. They are about embracing life as it is and finding joy in every moment, making not just for a longer life, but a life lived fully in every sense of the word.

Thus, imbibing insights from Sardinian living isn't just about eating what they eat or doing what they do. It also involves changing the way we think - pivoting from a goal-oriented, future-focused mindset to an encompassing, present-induced one.

This chapter, encapsulating the tranquility of a Sardinian's mind, truly helps us realize how simplifying our lives personally and professionally, learning to meditate in our daily tasks, and contemplating on the nature of contentment can silently lead us towards a healthy and prolonged life - the Sardinian way.

Emotional Balance and Health

After understanding the importance of diet, physical well-being, and social connections, it is crucial not to overlook another salient aspect: emotional wellness. The element of emotional stability plays a pivotal role in maintaining a balance between longevity and health. In the Blue Zones, including Sardinia, you'll find this is a vital cog in the wheel of lifelong health.

Emotional health is interconnected with physiological health. Our emotions can affect our immune system, cardiovascular health, and hormonal balance. Long-term emotional stress can lead to a myriad of health issues, including heart disease, digestive issues, sleep problems, weight gain, and memory disturbances.

However, the people in Blue Zones have found ways to counteract emotional stress and promote emotional health. They understand that maintaining an emotional balance is not about avoiding emotions. Rather, it's about acknowledging feelings–both positive and negative–and managing them effectively. That helps them stay healthier, happier, and ultimately, live longer.

Time-honored practices like mindfulness, meditation, prayer, and bonding with family and friends can drastically improve emotional health. In Sardinia, there's a strong emphasis on these practices. The community is closely-knit, families and friends are supportive, and there's a substantial respect for solitude and moments of quiet reflection.

A stable emotional state can also result in positive outlooks on life, acceptance, resilience, and even the ability to laugh at life's incongruities. Humor, in particular, has a significant role in Sardinian culture effective in stress reduction. It's common to find Sardinians aged 100 or more having roaring laughter-filled conversations with their friends and family.

Coping mechanisms also come into play when discussing emotional balance. Handling life's trials and tribulations with grace and acceptance forms part of the Sardinian way of life. Their lifestyle allows for the occasional hardships of life, letting them pass without a lasting negative impact on their emotional health.

Sardinians are known for their laid-back, stress-free lifestyle, which offers them the advantage of better emotional health. They've mastered the art of choosing actions that promote feelings of joy and happiness, and de-emphasize those that lead to stress or sadness.

Forgiveness is also celebrated in the Sardinian culture, along with a deep appreciation for the rhythm of life. Holding onto resentments, grudges, or negative feelings can be detrimental to emotional and physical health. Championing a spirit of understanding and forgiveness, Sardinians foster emotional stability and prevent the buildup of harmful emotions.

Also, Sardinians possess a clear sense of purpose in life. Having a sense of direction or a reason to get up in the morning, known as 'ikigai' in Japanese, enhances overall well-being and contributes to longer life expectancy. Whether it's looking after their grandchildren, tending to their gardens, or contributing to their communities, these purposes add meaning to their lives and drive them forward every day.

In an era when the modern world grapples with stress, anxiety, and depression, the people of Sardinia have retained their tradition of living emotionally balanced lives. Their appreciation for interpersonal connections, fun, forgiveness, purpose, and tranquility offers an antidote to the emotional stress rampant in many contemporary societies.

To sum up, the emotional balance present in the Blue Zones is multifaceted—stemming from strong community bonds, humor, an appreciation of life, healthy coping mechanisms, and a definite sense of purpose. Each of these factors complements the other, working in harmony to maintain emotional wellness.

More and more, science is beginning to validate these elements--underscoring that emotional balance and health can indeed contribute to longevity. As we unravel more about these aspects within the Blue Zones, integrating them into our lives can help us follow the path toward increased life expectancy and better health. Soulful nourishment can be just as important as physical nutrition.

Everything is intertwined. We simply can't separate the physical from the emotional. Our bodies react to how we feel, think, and behave. If we seek longevity and health, it's high time we took a look at how we handle our emotions and make necessary changes to ensure a balanced and healthy emotional state.

Perhaps the true secret to longevity goes beyond mere diet and physical activity. Perhaps it's also found in our hearts and minds—in the emotional wellness and balance that paints our everyday experiences with joyful color. As seen in Blue Zones like Sardinia, emotional health is undoubtedly an integral thread in the tapestry of a long, fulfilling life.

Chapter 6: Medical Insights and Healthcare

The intertwining relationship between the medical system, preventative healthcare practices, and a flourishing lifespan injects a layer of reasoning into understanding Sardinia's impressive longevity rates. A deep dive into Sardinian healthcare practices reveals a conscious approach that bridges modern medicine with traditional wisdom. This chapter will uncover how the medical ecosystem, grounded in both knowledge and compassion, nurtures longevity among the Sardinian populace. Emphasis is given to preventative measures and treatments utilized here, showing that prevention is indeed better than cure. We shall identify the integrative health approaches, combining techniques to heal not just the body, but also the mind and soul, thus delineating a holistic view of health. Furthermore, we will explore the synergy between early diagnosis, lifestyle modifications, natural remedies, and technology to shed light on how Sardinians continue to rule the roost in the longevity league. Unwrapping the vital role of medical insights and healthcare in Sardinia's longevity spectacle pinpoints the importance of a balanced healthcare system for sustained wellbeing.

Healthcare Practices in Sardinia

In Sardinia, healthcare practices, much like their dietary and social habits, are deeply rooted in their historical culture and local wisdom. The approach to healthcare is heavily human-centric, focusing more on preventive measures, traditional healing methods, and natural remedies rather than relying solely on modern medical technology.

One common feature of Sardinian healthcare is the regular use of local medicinal plants and herbs. This knowledge of local flora has been passed down through generations and has incorporated itself as a major part of Sardinian healthcare. The Sards use herbs such as helichrysum, mallow, and thyme, known for their various health benefits, including anti-inflammatory and antibacterial properties.

Another inherently Sardinian practice is prioritizing regular check-ups and health assessments. Sardinians do this not as a reactive measure to a health issue but as a routine preventive step. Regular health assessments are done to monitor health conditions and catch potential health threats early, enabling more effective management and treatment.

An interesting aspect of Sardinian healthcare practice is the influence of familial and communal support in health management. Families take an active role in caring for their sick or elder members at home, which often leads to more personalized and holistic care. In many cases, the community also plays a vital role in providing support and care, fostering a strong sense of belonging and overall mental health which, in turn, contributes to enhanced overall health.

Closely related to this is the considerate attention to mental health in Sardinia. It is seen as an integral part of overall wellbeing and is embedded in the Sardinian lifestyle through practices such as spending quality time with family, friends, engaging in daily physical activities, and maintaining spiritual practices. This integrated approach to health demonstrates that in Sardinia, health is viewed as a complete state of physical, mental, and social well-being, not merely the absence of disease or infirmity.

In addition to these practices, the use of traditional healing techniques is still prevalent in many parts of Sardinia. Practices such as plant-based remedies, body massages, and acupuncture have long stood the test of time. Despite advancements in modern medicine, they continue to co-exist, often complementary, side by side with it.

Another interesting practice is the emphasis on outdoor activities to manage and improve health, particularly mental health. With Sardinia's stunning natural landscapes, Sards often take walks, farm work or swim in the sea. These activities are considered therapeutic, promoting both physical fitness and mental tranquility.

One may argue that more than anything else, the Sardinians' attitude towards health and wellness could be the key to their extraordinary longevity. Sardinians seem to have a less stressful perspective towards life in general. They do not view ageing as something to be feared or fought against, but rather as a natural process to be accepted and embraced.

The Sardinian healthcare system is also structured to support this holistic approach. While it comprises modern hospitals and clinics, healthcare extends beyond these establishments. It is interwoven into social norms, cultural habits, and lifestyle choices, embodying a comprehensive approach that caters to holistic well-being.

This focus on preventative healthcare, combined with a sturdy social support network, a healthy diet, regular physical activities, and a positive mental outlook, all come together to form the secret recipe for the Sardinians' remarkable longevity.

Sardinians' approach to healthcare serves as a reminder that good health and longevity are not solely dependent on medical advancements and treatments as they are a product of lifestyle choices and cultural practices, suggesting that the key to longevity may not be found in a singular solution, but rather in a balanced way of life.

This human-centric and balanced approach to healthcare practiced in Sardinia might be seen as less technologically advanced compared to other parts of the world. Still, there's no denying the impressive result: longevity and, more importantly, quality of life and well-being.

Healthcare practices in Sardinia provide a refreshing perspective, a relaxed life outlook, and integrated health systems that bring modern and conventional medicine together. They are as much a testament to human adaptability and knowledge as they are a blueprint for other communities worldwide looking to improve overall health and lifespan.

In conclusion, while healthcare practices in Sardinia undoubtedly contribute towards their impressive longevity, it wasn't the only factor. Their approach to health and wellness is a fusion of several elements - a combination of their diet, social connections, lifestyle habits and the healthcare practices. This holistic approach offers a compelling alternative model for other communities to consider, not merely for longevity but for a life of quality and contentment.

Preventative Measures and Treatments

As we delve into the healthcare practices and preventative measures that contribute to Sardinia's reputation as a longevity hot spot, consider that health is not merely the absence of disease but a holistic state of well-being. Now, let's focus on the specific preventive measures and treatments that lie at the heart of this impressive longevity.

Sardinians, primarily those living in the rural Blue Zones, seldom wait for a health crisis before taking action. Growing up, they naturally incorporate healthy habits that safeguard them from many diseases such as heart disease, diabetes, and certain kinds of cancer.

One readily observable practice among the Sardinians is their regular engagement in physical activities. This doesn't necessitate rigorous high-impact workouts or pricey gym memberships. Instead, it's continuous and moderate activities like gardening, herding, or walking. Regular exercise enhances cardiovascular health, wards off obesity and its associated health complications, and strengthens muscles and bones, an essential consideration for aging populations to prevent falls and fractures.

A cornerstone of Sardinian preventative healthcare revolves around their dietary habits. Their predominantly plant-based diet rich in beans, whole grains, fruits, and vegetables provides ample vitamins, minerals, dietary fiber, and antioxidants that ward off disease by reducing inflammation and oxidative stress. Equally crucial is moderate consumption of animal products and red wine, which provides heart-healthy polyphenols.

Neither should we underestimate the therapeutic value of their traditional herbal medicine. For instance, the use of locally sourced herbs like Helichrysum, commonly used as an anti-inflammatory, and Thyme, believed to possess antiseptic properties. Utilized as treatments as much as preventative measures, these plant-based elixirs contribute towards maintaining a robust immune system.

The Sardinian approach to healthcare also considers mental health. Understanding the interconnectedness of physical and mental health, people living in these Blue Zones invest in maintaining strong social connections and partaking in community activities. This social participation isn't just for amusement - it staves off mental health conditions like depression and anxiety that can do severe damage if left untreated.

Furthermore, maintaining familial relationships in Sardinia is not just a question of social etiquette, but a health-preserving tradition. Growing old at home surrounded by family, both young and old, contributes to emotional health and a sense of purpose - key elements that have been linked to improved longevity.

Another important preventative measure is the promotion of stress management. Sardinians may work hard, but they also appreciate the value of leisure and relaxation. Regular downtime, naps, and the well-known Mediterranean tradition of 'La Passeggiata' - a leisurely communal walk at dusk – all play a role in managing stress levels and promoting overall health.

Sardinia's geographical isolation has led to a healthcare system largely focused on basic care rather than high-tech treatments. While this may seem like a disadvantage, there is a gentle irony to it. Rather than excessively focusing on high-cost reactive healthcare, Sardinians naturally gravitate towards low-cost preventative measures that ensure extended health and longevity.

Moreover, the healthcare system in Sardinia is equipped with excellent primary care, with a well-structured network of family doctors. Notably, these physicians are known to take a comprehensive approach to care, making house visits and prioritizing preventative care over high-tech treatments. They cultivate long-term relationships with their patients and pay heed to both physical and psychological symptoms.

It's also worth noting that Sardinians approach ailments with an amazing level of equanimity. This isn't indifference, but acceptance—recognizing that not all health conditions can be cured, but they can be managed with the correct attitude and treatment, thereby reducing unnecessary anxiety and stress.

In conclusion, several preventative measures and treatments play a role in Sardinia's impressive longevity. These range from those intertwined with daily life - such as dietary choices, physical activity, and social relationships - to those centered around traditional healthcare practices, herbal medicine, and stress management. Everything is interlinked, working in tandem to promote a robust health standard that sustains life well into old age.

Our exploration is far from over. As we move on to the next section, we will take a more in-depth look at the holistic aspect of this entire picture and see how integrative health approaches play a significant role in Sardinian longevity. By understanding these practices, we can tease apart the secrets of these Blue Zones and maybe even apply them to our own lives.

Integrative Health Approaches

Shifting our perspective to the realm of health medicine, we'll see that in Sardinia, the approach to healthcare is distinctive. While they obviously do not discredit modern medicine and its benefits, they lean heavily towards integrative healthcare approaches. This leans toward a more holistic approach to health, bridging the gap between conventional medicine and natural healing traditions.

The integrative health approach is considered one of the keys to the centuries-long health and vitality of Sardinians. This system of healthcare brings together different facets of medical therapies, combining them to address the full range of physical, emotional, mental, social health, and wellness. So how does it work exactly?

An integrative approach to health focuses on the patient as a whole rather than just on the disease. It values the patient-practitioner relationship and sets a premium on patient-centered care. In Sardinia, it's not uncommon for healthcare practitioners to spend considerable time with patients, understanding their lifestyle, diet, habits, and emotional wellbeing. This is because each of these factors is regarded as considerably impactful on overall health.

One essential component of this approach is the use of herbal medicines and natural remedies. Sardinians have been using medicinal plants and herbs for centuries, and these traditional remedies play a significant role in their healthcare. The bushes of Mediterranean maquis, the forests high in the mountains, and the fertile plains of the island are rich sources of healing herbs such as myrtle, thyme, rosemary, and fennel. These are often used in the preparation of food, drinks, poultices, and infusions to treat common complaints and maintain health.

Another essential aspect of the integrative health approach in Sardinia is their customary physical activities. Manual labor, whether it be farming, fishing, or herding, plays a significant role in keeping Sardinians active. It serves as a natural form of exercise that contributes to their cardiovascular health and optimal weight management.

Emotional and mental health are also prioritized in this integrative approach. Strong family ties and a sense of community provide Sardinians with emotional support, and many centenarians attribute their longevity to their happy and stress-free life. Activities such as socializing with family, friends, and neighbors, storytelling, singing, dancing, and playing traditional games contribute to their emotional health and mental well-being.

Another key element in the Sardinian integrative healthcare model is their traditional diet. On the island, mealtime is a reason for celebration and socialization. The traditional Sardinian diet, centered on whole foods such as vegetables, fruits, lean proteins, whole grains, and healthy fats, plays a significant role in their good health and longevity.

Of course, Sardinia isn't immune to modern-day medical practices. Traditional healthcare remedies coexist with modern medicine, and Sardinians regularly seek professional healthcare for preventive measures and treatment. What makes the difference is a distinct preference for natural, less invasive methods whenever possible.

In Sardinia, it's crucial to strike a balance. The synergy of prevenction-oriented lifestyle, traditional remedies, and modern science is viewed as the optimal integrative model for health. This balance is a key part of the puzzle explaining Sardinian longevity.

Sardinians also heavily practice prevention. A strong focus is set on lifestyle choices that prevent the onset of disease, rather than merely treating the symptoms once they occur. Regular check-ups and screenings are common, with preventative measures such as healthy eating and active living being a part and parcel of everyday life.

It is important to bear in mind that these health measures are rooted in centuries-old traditions, passed down from generation to generation. This inherited wisdom has been integrated into Sardinian life in a way that makes it an intrinsic part of their culture.

One could surmise that the Sardinian approach to health and longevity is an excellent illustration of integrative healthcare at its finest. It marries the best of modern medicine with time-tested natural remedies and lifestyle choices to promote health, well-being, and longevity. The emphasis is not just on living long, but on living well, considering all dimensions of one's being. In the end, the Sardinian longevity secret may not be such a secret after all: balance in life might be the key we've been searching for.

In the next chapter, we'll delve deeper into the Sardinian culture, revealing intimate aspects of living through personal stories, wisdom, and life lessons from those who have made it to the incredible milestone of one hundred years. Such testimonies will afford us a closer look at the practices and beliefs that have functioned as a blueprint to longevity in Sardinian society.

Chapter 7: Stories from the Elders

Diving into Chapter 7, we delve into the real treasure chest of Sardinia—the stories from its elders. Their fascinating narratives, a blend of history and wisdom, unveil profound secrets of longevity. It's not just about a diet rich in local, organic foods, or a sequestered terrain that seems to lend itself to the 'natural gym' of everyday activities. It's the unwritten stories, the oral traditions passed down through generations, offering invaluable life lessons and personal perspectives on living a long, fulfilling life. Grandparents, nonagenarians and centenarians, provide a lively commentary on lifestyle practices, attitudes and the very ethos of Sardinian society. Interspersed with anecdotes, their narratives elucidate how love for the land, close-knit families, and active social engagements form the triangular pillar of Sardinian longevity. Here, the concept of age isn't just a number, but rather a badge of honor, a testament to strength, endurance and wisdom earned through years lived and experiences gathered. For many of these elders, longevity isn't so much about the goal of reaching an impressive age, but rather a happy by-product of a life lived in harmony with nature, community, and self.

Interviews with Centenarians

As we explore the stories of Sardinia's centenarians, it's refreshing to see that their narratives are not burdened by rigid regimens or complicated formulas. Instead, they convey an essence of simplicity, balance, and natural connectedness that gives everyday life a sense of joy and purpose.

One of the centenarians we interviewed is Marianna, a 103-year-old woman from a small village in Barbagia. She credits her longevity to a life of hard work, a simple diet abundant with fresh local produce, and strong family connections. Marianna's life peeks into the consistent themes that we've encountered in earlier chapters - a nourishing diet, a working lifestyle, and a close-knit community.

Next, we met with a sprightly 102-year-old man named Euris. He generously attributed his longevity to frequent walks in the surrounding hills, the crisp clean air and the level of peace attainable here. These observations once again echo the important roles of physical activity and a serene environment in the well-being of Sardinia's long-lived residents.

We also had the honor of speaking with a delightful 108-year-old lady named Stella. Humor twinkled in her eyes as she declared wine and song were secrets to her long life. She stated that daily glass of homemade wine and regular participation in village celebrations kept her spirit young. This fascinating conversation underscored the longevity advantage of moderate alcohol consumption and social engagement, particularly involving music and dance.

Our conversation with Vincenzo, a centenarian shepherd who spent most of his life herding sheep in the Sardinian highlands, revealed another important aspect of the Sardinian lifestyle. He highlighted the gratification derived from meaningful work and following an ancient way of life. From Vincenzo's perspective, sticking to long-established routines and leading an active lifestyle underpin his extraordinary longevity.

We traveled to Seulo, a village renowned for a high concentration of centenarians, to interview 101-year-old

Anna. Anna expressed the significance of maintaining close family ties, suggesting that the love and support from family members contribute to her emotional well-being and health. Anna's insights provide a testament to the critical role of family and social ties in prolonging life expectancy.

Further, we had an enlightening conversation with Natalina, a lively 100-year-old. She emphasized the importance of a positive mindset, expressing no attention to her age whatsoever. Natalina's longevity secret underlined the fact that age is more than just a number, but also a state of mind.

Each centenarian we met offered unique insights into the Sardinian way of life that contributes to their extended lifespan. However, despite the differing perspectives, a number of consistent themes were apparent. A moderate, balanced diet; an active lifestyle; a strong sense of community; and a positive mindset repeatedly cropped up in their stories.

While these themes resonate with the scientific understanding of what contributes to longevity, these centenarians' stories highlight the importance of how these elements are naturally integrated into daily living. They demonstrate that it is less about implementing drastic lifestyle changes, and more about fostering an environment and a culture that naturally embody these longevity-enhancing factors.

Looking at our lives through the lens of these centenarians provides a fresh perspective. The simplicity of their lifestyle contrasts strikingly with the complexity and hectic pace of modern living. Yet, it calls us to reflect on how we can cultivate similar patterns of behavior in our own lives and embed those healthful habits into our daily routines.

These conversations with Sardinian centenarians serve as personal reminders of the potency of engaging with our natural environment, socializing within our community, maintaining a balanced diet, and preserving a positive mindset. These factors are intimately intertwined, constituting a holistic approach to longevity which supersedes disjointed or compartmentalized health behaviors.

It is also clear that the benefits of this lifestyle extend beyond mere longevity. The centenarians expressed a contentment and satisfaction with life, highlighting an important distinction between simply living longer and living well. Their stories embody a deep sense of wellness that extends across physical, mental, and emotional dimensions.

Admittedly, recreating a Sardinian lifestyle in other parts of the world poses challenges due to cultural, climatic, and geographical differences. However, the fundamental principles promoting longevity are universally applicable. More than prescriptive guidelines, they call for a shift in the approach to life, underscoring the importance of balance, enjoyment, social engagement, and harmony with nature.

The wisdom shared by the Sardinian centenarians elucidates the factors contributing to a long and fulfilling life. By integrating these principles into our lives, we can start to create our personal blue zones, cultivating an environment that supports not just longevity, but also the quality of life.

Living beyond one's centenary year is a feat not accomplished by many. However, it is one that offers valuable insights. On taking inspiration from these centenarians, it would seem the secrets are clear – balance, simplicity, hard work, close-knit communities, and a positive state of mind are the cornerstones of a long and healthy life.

Wisdom and Life Lessons

The average longevity of Sardinian centenarians can be traced back through their stories, experiences, wisdom, and life lessons handed down from generation to generation. These lessons aren't necessarily structured teachings or immediately evident. Still, they can be found simmering below the surface of daily interactions, shaping a way of life conducive to physical and emotional well-being.

On the surface, it may seem that the villagers live the way they do wholly unaware of the complexities behind their habits, practices, and customs. Yet in the simplicity of their everyday living, residents of Sardinia manage to capture the essence of longevity. It's the principle of living harmoniously with oneself, the community, and the environment.

One commonly shared piece of wisdom in Sardinian culture is the importance of community ties and unity. Villagers emphasize mutual cooperation, support, and above all, respect for one another, irrespective of age or status. Everyone enjoys a strong sense of belonging and shared identity, which leads to lower stress levels and longer, healthier lives.

An understanding of the essence of daily work is another important life lesson. It's not seen as a means to an end, but an intrinsic part of life contributing to physical health, emotional well-being, and a sense of purpose. Work is not limited to making a living but extends to working in the gardens, on the lands, and at home, cultivating a non-sedentary lifestyle that contributes to longevity.

Nutrition-wise, Sardinians' wisdom is deeply rooted in respect for local, seasonal, and minimally processed food. They treasure their locally grown crops, with a predilection for beans, whole grains, fruits, and vegetables. This reverence for nature's bounty, encapsulated in their dietary habits, can serve as an instructive lesson in sustaining human health and environmental balance.

But nutrition is not merely an act of physical sustenance. The act of consuming food is coupled with the principle of enjoyment. Meals are not hurried affairs; instead, they are savored, often in the company of others, reinforcing social ties and psychological satisfaction.

Another guiding principle in Sardinian culture is spiritual and emotional well-being. Sardinians value contentment, mindfulness, and balance in life. They celebrate with music, laughter, and wine, offering profound life lessons on the importance of joy, pleasure, and relaxation in longevity.

Importantly, respect and care for the elderly run deep within Sardinian society, a lesson in itself. Elders are integrated into family life and are viewed as bearers of wisdom and experience. They play active roles in raising grandchildren, instilling cultural values, and contributing to community life.

Healthcare in Sardinia is not just about medical treatments. Their approach leans more towards prevention than cure. They rely largely on natural remedies, dietary practices, and traditional healing techniques. In essence, they practice integrative healing, which brings about whole-system wellness.

Overall, the Sardinian philosophy of life revolves around a mixture of elements that contribute to longevity: hard work, but not overwork; respect for nature and its rhythms; a diet that nourishes; emotional balance nurtured through strong social connections; and the valuing of all stages of life. These are the life lessons weaved into the fabric of Sardinian life.

In embracing these lessons, we're called not only to enact certain behaviors but also to absorb deeper values: respect for community, appreciation for nature, balance, modesty, and, importantly, contentment. Herein lie lessons that resonate beyond Sardinia, providing guidance for anyone seeking to live a healthier, longer life.

The wisdom of Sardinia may not be contained in the volumes of books, but rather in the rhythm of life that pulses through the veins of its inhabitants — in their fields, homes, gatherings, and spirituality. So, the best way to learn from Sardinia isn't merely to study their practices, but to immerse yourself in their attitude towards life.

In this world of seemingly rapid advancement and change, Sardinian lifestyle and values act as a reminder of the timeless wisdom that can guide us towards healthier, more fulfilling, and yes, possibly longer, lives that embody quality and contentment. Applying these lessons is more than a just method to longer life. It's a gateway to a life lived in harmony and balance, to a life well-lived.

Personal Perspectives on Longevity

We've been fascinated by the vivid tales, wise anecdotes, and enriching life experiences shared by Sardinia's centenarians. Their stories provide an invaluable source mark, a subjective and deeply human standpoint on achieving longevity. What follows in this section is a compilation of these personal perspectives.

One notable common thread is the emphasis on diet and physical activity. "We eat what our land gives us. We work hard in the fields. That's our secret," said Antonio, a sprightly 101-year-old. Such simple statements resonate with the comprehensive research that underscores the role of these two factors in contributing to a longer life.

More than just meal content, dining rituals also emerged as a component of their longevity. Sharing meals with loved ones and taking time to enjoy food slowly can't be overstated in its significance. "We've always taken meals together, as a family," Lucia, 102, shared. "We talk, laugh, argue... the food tastes better that way."

In addition to diet and activity, preserving a high level of interaction with family and community was another strong theme. The elderly were not segregated or marginalized in any way. Maria, 100, put it beautifully, "We are old in age but not in spirit. We stay active by helping with the grandchildren, contributing to the family, and participating in community events."

Socially allocated roles for those in their golden years often involve passing down wisdom, teaching younger ones skills, mentoring, and mediating in conflicts. Giovanni, 103, sees his role as a guardian of traditions, "Keeping our culture alive, I tell stories to the younger ones. That's what keeps me young."

Surprisingly, it isn't just about the physical activities or social participation, but also the embrace of a slower pace of life. "We take time to enjoy life's simple pleasures - a good meal, a beautiful sunset, companionship. It's not about living fast, but living fully," said Paolo, who celebrated his 105th birthday recently.

From a mental health perspective, these centenarians carry a unique outlook on life and show an amazing ability to stay centered, poised, and maintain perspective in the face of adversity. "Troubles come and go, life is full of ebbs and flows. One has to stay calm and carry on," mused Carmen, 104.

Another significant element highlighted by many was their relationship with nature. The majority of centenarians have spent a lifetime working land, taking care of animals, or fishing. They underlined the substantial role that an active life in outdoors plays both on a physical and mental level. Grazia, 106, explained, "Nature is my therapy. In the fields, I lose all my worries."

The spiritual lens through which they view life also appears to contribute to longevity. "The faith has always kept me strong, given me a sense of purpose and reassured me during hard times," confided Rosa, aged 101. Whether it's through organized religion or private spirituality, a belief in a higher power appears to be a significant factor.

What's evident in these candid revelations is that the secret of longevity doesn't fall into a single formula. It's an amalgamation of numerous elements - balanced diets, strong community ties, robust mental health, and a fulfilling role in society. Embracing hardship and living harmoniously with the natural world also play major parts.

Lessons from these centenarians suggest that longevity is not a mere biophysical phenomenon. It is intimately woven into the island's culture, societal structures, environment, and spiritual beliefs. It's about maintaining an inner equilibrium, being resilient yet serene, living vibrantly, and staying engaged with life.

As we close this chapter about personal perspectives, we suggest that you pause for a moment. Digest these insights and examine their implications for your own lifetime. And remember, living longer isn't merely about counting the years, but more about making those years count.

And as we move to our next chapter 'Beyond Sardinia - The Global Blue Zones', we will be venturing into a comparative exploration of how the intriguing phenomenon of longevity manifests itself in other parts of the globe.

Subjectivity adds color to the scientific reality painted by objectivity. The personal tales told by Sardinia's centenarians enrich our understanding of longevity, transforming it from sheer statistics into a tangible, human experience. It gives the phenomenon a face, a story, a voice - unmistakably real and inspiringly familiar.

Chapter 8: Beyond Sardinia - The Global Blue Zones

As we venture beyond Sardinia, we're inevitably drawn toward an exploration of the wider world of Blue Zones. Numerous other regions around the globe nurture societies that boast remarkable longevity, each with its own unique combination of dietary, lifestyle, and social factors that contribute to the health and vitality of its residents. A comparative analysis of these Blue Zones uncovers interesting parallels, yet, also highlighting significant differences that can be attributed to the variety of cultural contexts. From the lush Nicoya Peninsula in Costa Rica to the serene island of Okinawa in Japan, longevity isn't confined to a single demographic or geographic profile, but flourishes under diverse conditions bolstered by nuanced, yet strikingly consistent determinants. The collective wisdom gleaned from these regions offers invaluable lessons and implications, not merely for those aiming to enhance their own longevity, but for societies worldwide seeking sustainable strategies to improve public health and overall well-being.

Comparisons with Other Blue Zones

Before we delve into comparisons, lest we forget that Sardinia distinguishes itself as the first recognized Blue Zone, the point of origin of this concept. But, the world is vast, and longevity has other addressable ties in places like Okinawa, Japan, Loma Linda, California, and the highland villages of Ikaria, Greece, and the Nicoya Peninsula, Costa Rica.

In Okinawa, the archipelago of Japan, people are blessed with longer lives. Much like Sardinia, Okinawans attribute their longevity to a healthy diet, abundant in local produce. However, unlike the Sardinian reliance on the Mediterranean diet, Okinawans' reliance on a plant-based diet primarily featuring sweet potatoes, soy products, and a diversity of vegetables is noteworthy. They also share a sense of community and life imbued with purpose, but the spiritual form of it differs from the Christian beliefs predominantly seen in Sardinia.

Conversely, in Loma Linda, California, the lifestyle and mindset have set this town apart. The longevity observed among the Seventh-Day Adventists in Loma Linda can be linked to their religiously grounded principles on diet, exercise, and rest. Their vegetarian diet, which symbolizes respect for the human body as a 'temple of the Holy Spirit,' deviates from Sardinia's dietary habits but shares the core understanding of the body's health as essential.

Moving on to the highland villages of Ikaria, Greece, the focus is less on work and more on socializing, celebrating life, and taking the day slowly—an aspect shared with the Sardinians. Their Mediterranean diet aligns closely with Sardinia's, with a focus on fruits, vegetables, whole grains, and olive oil. Ikarians also highly value socializing and integrating physical activity into daily life.

Further south, the Nicoya Peninsula in Costa Rica has its unique Blue Zone. Like Sardinia, Nicoyans value strong social networks and dedicate time to live a slower pace of life. Nevertheless, their diet is different, dominated by beans, corn, squash, tropical fruits, and a specific kind of tortilla, underlying the significance of a balanced, healthy diet to obtain a pleasurable, long life.

Despite their geographical and cultural disparities, Blue Zones seem to share some common themes that contribute to their longevity. The most prominent among these shared elements is the significance placed on diet where locally sourced, and predominantly plant-based foods are prioritized.

Another common feature shared by these regions is the emphasis on maintaining strong family ties and a vibrant social life. This sense of community has been linked time and again to improved mental well-being and, consequently, longer lifespans, whether it's the closely-knit families of Sardinia or the 'moai' groups in Okinawa.

Active living, which involves integrating physical activities into daily routines, is another characteristic seen across these regions. In Blue Zones, physical activity isn't just limited to a workout routine but is embedded in daily life, from Sardinian shepherds tending to their flock to Okinawans practicing Tai Chi.

But it's not all about the external. Across the board, Blue Zones indicate that emotional well-being is just as important as physical health. From the Costa Ricans' 'Pura Vida' philosophy to the contentment of the Greek elders, Blue Zone populations appear to have cracked the code on maintaining emotional balance.

The way health and healthcare are perceived and addressed is yet another shared characteristic among the Blue Zones. They generally lean towards prevention over cure, with an emphasis on natural remedies and holistic healing.

These comparisons reveal that no matter which Blue Zone we venture into, the secrets of longevity seem overlapping yet distinct. The interconnectedness between a balanced diet, physical activity, emotional well-being, strong social ties, and caring healthcare systems has been deeply rooted in the heart of each Blue Zone community's daily life. So what are the global implications?

The idea is simple. The Blue Zone approach seems to imply that longevity isn't just about personal habits or genetic disposition. It's about the environments we cultivate, both within ourselves and in our societies. Through an examination of common threads such as diet, social structures, active living, spiritual outlook, and healthcare practices, Blue Zones provide a longevity blueprint for the rest of the world.

Even though we might live in radically different contexts from the inhabitants of these Blue Zones, we can glean cherished lessons about leading healthier, longer, and happier lives. It's not just about copying diet plans or exercise routines. Instead, it's more about fostering an environment around us that naturally encourages better physical, mental, and social health.

On the next level, these findings raise profound questions about our current habits and lifestyle choices. They challenge the prevailing global norms on food, family, work, leisure, and medicine, propelling us to rethink our ways and adapt patterns that promote long, healthy, and satisfying lives.

Indeed, by examining such different Blue Zones—each with its unique cultural, geographical, and societal settings—we can find our way to cherry-pick best practices, adapt them as per our circumstances, and sow the seeds of our own Blue Zones. The aspiration is not to match their life spans inch by inch but to embrace an ethos that champions well-being and longevity in its own right.

Commonalities and Differences

We've spent a good deal of time delving into the many aspects of the Sardinian lifestyle. We've unraveled the mysteries of their diet, active cultural practices, cherished family and community ties and their unique and holistic medical insights. Their profound spiritual and emotional wellbeing and the invaluable wisdom of their elders have been extensively detailed. Now, let's shift gears slightly to compare how these elements hold up against practices from other blue zones around the world.

Firstly, it's worth mentioning that the lessons we've learned from the Sardinian blue zones are not unique. Interestingly, the centenarian populations in other blue zones across the world, such as Okinawa in Japan and Loma Linda in California, share many commonalities with the Sardinians. These consist of a predominantly plant-based diet, rich social and community interactions, habitual physical activity, and a deep sense of purpose in life.

However, while these communities share some broad lifestyle patterns, their individual approaches can be quite distinct. For instance, the diet in Okinawa, is characterized by a high consumption of sweet potatoes and tofu, while Loma Linda's Seventh-day Adventists are known for a vegetarian or vegan diet. This gives us a clue that there's no one-size-fits-all approach to longevity; rather, a combination of beneficial lifestyle habits, cultural values, and traditional practices.

Blue Zones, despite being geographically dispersed and culturally diverse, seem to converge at a set of foundational principles that drive longevity. Central to these is the accent on natural, balanced, and wholesome diets that favor local and unprocessed ingredients.

Similarities extend beyond just dietary practices. The emphasis on family, social ties, and community involvement is another shared trait among these longevity hotspots. In Okinawa, it's the familial moais or supportive social networks while in Loma Linda, it's deeply ingrained religious community ties that provide psychological support and shared values.

The integration of physical activity into everyday life is also recognized as a key contributor to increased lifespan. However, the form of the activity varies greatly with the activities being woven into the fabric of daily living, rather than being an afterthought or chore. Sardinians count their pastoral and agricultural life while Okinawans are well-known for their Tai Chi practices.

However, these commonalities notwithstanding, there are stark differences in how each of these societies approach life. It could be the spiritual integration of the Seventh-day Adventists, or the prominence given to continuous learning and purposeful life even in old age by the Okinawans.

The medical practices adopted across the different Blue Zones also show distinct contrasts. While Sardinia favours a more organic approach backed by traditional wisdom, Okinawan longevity is often associated with the Japanese healthcare system that focuses on regular medical check-ups and treatments.

Even amidst the differences, a central theme of a mind-body-spirit balance resonates across all the Blue Zones. Emotional balance and spiritual contentment are shown to play a critical role in addition to physical well-being.

While many commonalities emerge, we must acknowledge the uniqueness of each Blue Zone. Their rich cultural legacies are shaped and evolved over time to cater to their specific geographic and societal conditions. Yet, in spite of the differences and nuances, they all testify to a universal truth - that it is indeed possible to live a long, fulfilling life.

Each Blue Zone holds valuable lessons in longevity, but it's also important to recognize the uniqueness of each zone. Sardinia, with its Mediterranean influence, pastoral lifestyle, close-knit communities, and holistic health practices gives a unique flavor to the concept of longevity, as do the eccentricities of Okinawa, Loma Linda, and others.

In essence, the crux of understanding these Blue Zones lies not just in their shared traits, but also in their differences. It is these variances that provide valuable insights into the multifaceted secrets of longevity, revealing that different paths can lead to the same goal: a long, fruitful life.

In the next chapter, we'll delve into how we can apply these lessons from the Sardinian and other Blue Zones to our own lives. It's one thing to theorize about living a long life, but quite another to put it into practice. Will the idyllic lifestyle translate to the urban jungle? Stick around to find out.

Global Implications and Lessons

As we've journeyed through Sardinia and other well-known Blue Zones, drawing comparisons and assessing unique patterns of longevity, myriad global implications have risen to the surface—proof that the world has a lot to learn from these longevity-inclined regions. The overarching lesson is clear: habits matter, and adopting healthier cultural norms can positively influence not just personal longevity, but also global health metrics.

For instance, one of the starkest differences we noted was the strong culture of physical activity intrinsic to Sardinian life.

Here, physical movement isn't a chore, it's a natural part of living—an outlook that has resulted in low obesity rates and improved cardiovascular health. This suggests a powerful lesson for more sedentary societies, where structured exercise routines might be replaced, or at least supplemented with, more passive, habitual physical movement.

Then, of course, we have the Sardinian diet—one that bursts with fresh, simple, and largely plant-based produce. Certain widespread health issues, such as heart disease and diabetes, have been closely tied to poor diet choices. By centering plant-based, unprocessed foods and whole grains—as is the norm in Sardinian homes—we can globally counteract some of these pernicious health concerns.

The prominence of communal relationships and familial bonds in Sardinia has profound implications for coping with mental health issues worldwide. Social isolation is a growing concern, especially in urbanized societies where individualism often overshadows community spirit. By fortifying social structures and fostering strong relationships, we can build emotional resilience and counteract the mental health strain currently plaguing many societies.

Sardinian spirituality and its interplay with emotional well-being also offer important lessons. The emphasis on mindfulness, contentment, and gratitude represent a stark contrast with hyper-materialistic cultures often marred by relentless pursuit of wealth and success. This misaligned focus can result in chronic stress, fatigue, and mental illnesses.

Considering healthcare, the integrative approach seen in Sardinia emphasizes prevention over cure, a lesson many systems obsessed with curing diseases can take note of. A holistic approach which encompasses mental, physical, and social aspects of health creates a more balanced and effective healthcare structure.

While global implications abound, a key takeaway is that no one-size-fits-all solution to longevity exists. The Sardinian lifestyle, influenced by its unique environment, history, and traditions, has forged a thriving culture of longevity that can't be packaged and exported as is.

Yet, Sardinia's blueprint is valuable as inspiration and guide to adapt and try in different societies. They serve as proof that longevity isn't solely dictated by genetics—one's environment and lifestyle play significant roles too.

The case of Sardinia isn't isolated either. The lifestyle patterns and underlying principles of other Blue Zones like Okinawa, Japan, and Loma Linda, USA, reinforce lessons learned from Sardinia. Although these zones have distinct cultures, similar threads bind them—natural physical activity, plant-based diets, robust social structures, and an overall balance of well-being.

Even outside Blue Zones, regions that incorporate similar lifestyle elements are witnessing improved health metrics. This suggests that these Blue Zones are analogues for healthful living, providing lessons applicable to communities globally.

There's also a clear signal for policymakers and public health experts that societal structures and norms play a massive role in determining health outcomes. Blue Zones offer a prototype of how societies can structure physical, social, and cultural ecosystems to facilitate healthier, longer lives.

Finally, we must acknowledge that changes won't occur overnight. Cultural shifts take time and persistence, yet the benefits are worthwhile. By adopting Blue Zone lessons into individual behaviors, policy initiatives, and community endeavors, we can make meaningful strides towards improved global health and increased longevity.

In conclusion, this journey into the heart of Blue Zones shouldn't be seen as exploration of foreign, exotic lands with mystical secrets to long life. Rather, it's a deeper inquiry into how our everyday choices—what we eat, how we move, our social interactions, and our approach to healthcare—have profound implications on our longevity. That's the most significant global lesson we must take away from Sardinia and other Blue Zones.

Chapter 9: Applying Sardinian Wisdom

Transitioning from a global exploration of blue zones, we now turn our focus towards practical application of lessons learned. The key to healthier living lies within the lifestyle choices we make every day, and the Sardinian model presents a practical blueprint we can borrow. Embracing a diet rich in local and Mediterranean-inspired whole foods not only contributes to physical health but also promotes sustainable living with minimal environmental impact. Another essential aspect lies in cultivating strong family and community bonds, which has far-reaching positive effects on mental well-being. Importantly, leading an active lifestyle, integrating regular physical activities, and maintaining a positive outlook on life are also powerful agents of longevity. However, it's critical to note that creating your own blue zone doesn't simply mean replicating the Sardinian way of life; it requires thoughtfully adapting these practices to your cultural context and personal circumstances. We'll further delve into the potential challenges one might encounter in attempting this transformation, such as dealing with modern societal pressures that may contradict these healthful practices, and how best to negotiate them for lasting success.

Practical Tips for Healthier Living

After a thorough exploration of Sardinia and unveiling its secrets to a long and healthy life, it's only fitting we compile the wisdom into practical tips for healthier living. The journey has been enlightening, peppered with fascinating tales, delicious recipes, engaging activities, and above all, the simplicity of Sardinian lifestyle.

Perhaps the most iconic element of the Sardinian lifestyle is the traditional Mediterranean diet. This widespread dietary pattern mainly emphasizes whole, unprocessed foods. These include seasonal fruits and vegetables, whole grains, legumes, fish, and extra virgin olive oil, accompanied by moderate consumption of red wine. Incorporating these elements into your everyday meals can make a massive difference in your overall health.

Equally significant is the culture of physical activity woven into the fabric of Sardinian life. Daily physical chores, whether they are related to farming, shepherding, or housekeeping, contribute significantly to keeping the Sardinians active. It's not about hitting the gym; it's about consistent, natural movement. We are encouraged to find opportunities in our daily routine to move - walking, gardening, cycling, or even standing instead of sitting can make a positive impact.

Meal-sharing and communal dining play enormous roles in Sardinian culture. Mealtimes are not just about eating; they're about sharing experiences, forming and strengthening social ties. Make an effort to eat at least one meal a day in the company of your loved ones. Social connections are crucial for mental wellness and have a profound impact on our overall health trajectory.

Speaking of mental wellness, the practice of mindfulness plays a big role in Sardinian culture. This can involve quiet reflection, meditation, or simply taking the time to enjoy beautiful sceneries and live in the moment. Incorporate a practice of mindfulness in your daily routine; it's a simple yet highly effective path to emotional balance.

The intergenerational connection is another worth noting aspect of life in Sardinia. Respect for the elderly and fostering relationships between the older and younger generations contributes significantly to the mental health of all involved. It is known that such interactions often lead to a heightened sense of purpose for the elders while providing a stable and loving environment for the younger generation. Engaging with family members of different generations can contribute to emotional enrichment.

Adopt the Sardinian inclination towards minimalism - a simple life is often a happier one. A focused life with less clutter, whether material or emotional, contributes to a mentally healthier lifestyle. Reducing unnecessary possessions and emotional baggage boosts your overall well-being.

Embrace positivity and laugh often. Sardinians are known for their love of life and humor. Laughter is a well-recognized stress buster, a natural medicine, and it's contagious too. Look for joy and humor in daily life.

Sardinians have a tendency for resilience and a generally optimistic outlook on life. Cultivating a positive mental attitude and resilience helps you cope with life's challenges. This is indeed synonymous with healthier living and longevity.

The practice of herbal remedies is popular in Sardinia. While it is not an encouragement to toss out conventional medicine, there's potential value in considering the benefits of herbal and botanical remedies alongside professional medical advice.

Encourage biodiversity around you. The relationship between Sardinians and their land demonstrates a respect towards nature, thereby encouraging biodiversity and sustainability. This respect for nature goes hand in hand with the healthier nutritional choices Sardinians make.

Let's not overlook the practice of an afternoon nap, or a siesta. This tradition might seem like a luxury, but it has a lot to do with the reduced instances of heart disease in Sardinia. Short, restful breaks during the day can reduce stress and boost productivity.

Sleep quality holds utmost importance in maintaining a healthier life. Aim for a good night's sleep - seven to eight hours is ideal. Maintain a consistent sleep-wake cycle, and implement a relaxing bedtime routine to wind down for the day.

In conclusion, a longer, healthier life isn't about one factor; it's about a complete lifestyle that includes a balanced diet, physical activity, socialisation, sleep, and above all, a positive outlook towards life.

As we venture to creating our own blue zones, these principles offer a roadmap to a healthier and longer life. It's never too late, or too early, to start making positive changes in your life for the sake of your well-being.

Creating Your Own Blue Zone

Incorporating the principles of Blue Zones into our lives might seem challenging at first glance, but the benefits can be substantial. This chapter will outline the process you can follow to transform your communities and personal lifestyle habits to emulate those found in recognized Blue Zones. The metaphor of creating a "Blue Zone" should not be misunderstood. You can't literally turn the geographic location in which you reside into a longevity hotspot. What you can do, however, is apply the key principles and practices found in true Blue Zones to cultivate health and longevity in your personal life.

First, let's begin with the physical components. Exercise, particularly in the form of everyday activities, is central to a Blue Zone lifestyle. Recognized Blue Zones feature environmental characteristics that encourage regular physical activity, such as walkable communities. It's important to modify your living area, where possible, to maximize the need for simple, regular physical activity. Perhaps this means choosing an apartment that requires climbing stairs, or incorporating walking or biking into your daily commute. The goal is to seamlessly integrate exercise into your daily routine, rather than regarding it as a separate, often neglected, task.

Diet is another critical component. Blue Zones are typically characterized by a plant-based diet, with an emphasis on fresh, organic, and locally sourced produce. It might not be possible to completely replicate Sardinian or Okinawan cuisines, for example, but integrating more fruits, vegetables, whole grains, and legumes into your diet, while reducing the amount of processed foods, can significantly enhance your health and longevity.

Moreover, adopting the practice of consuming smaller portions and not eating until you're full can also be beneficial. Experience the Sardinian practice of eating your largest meal early and limiting dinner to small, light portions. The intention is not only to nourish your body but also to cultivate a relationship with food that is balanced and mindful.

Mental well-being and stress management form another cornerstone of Blue Zone living. This includes regular social interaction, as well as practices promoting mindfulness and relaxation. While each person's approach to mental well-being will be highly individual, basics may include frequent socializing with friends and family, involvement in community activities, daily meditation or other relaxation exercises, and consistency in getting a good night's sleep.

One distinctive element of Blue Zones is the prevalence of strong, supportive communities. You can imitate this by nurturing close family ties, fostering supportive friendships, and getting involved in organizations that resonate with your values. Remember, the aim isn't to amass a large number of acquaintances; rather, the focus should be on cultivating deep, enriching relationships.

Many of us unknowingly lead isolating lives, constantly plugged into technology and disconnected from the people around us. We can learn from Blue Zone communities the importance of being more present and engaged in our interactions with others. These connections can become lifelines, providing emotional support, reducing stress and promoting longevity.

While you may not be able to fully recreate the context of a Blue Zone, you can apply principles from these areas in a meaningful way. One of those principles is taking time to unwind. This can take many forms, from taking a short nap after a meal, maintaining a hobby that relaxes you, or simply setting aside quiet time each day. The key is to find balance between productive work and restful, peaceful states of mind.

It's also important to note that Blue Zones aren't only about diet and exercise, they also place a profound emphasis on a sense of purpose. Having reason to get up in the morning is a very powerful thing. It could be your job, a hobby, community service, or your family - purpose is highly individual but crucial for longevity. Purpose-driven living promotes happiness, fulfillment, and ultimately, longer, healthier lives.

Remember, change does not happen overnight. Transitioning towards a Blue Zone way of life is a gradual process, requiring some experimentation and adjustments along the way. The key is to start with small, manageable changes and stay consistent. Over time, these efforts can improve your well-being and potentially your lifespan as well.

In concluding, creating your own Blue Zone doesn't mean moving to Sardinia or Okinawa. It's about making a conscious effort to adopt aspects of their wholesome lifestyles. It involves transforming physical environments, shifting mindset, creating mindful eating habits, nurturing purposeful relationships, and living a life filled with purpose.

Although it might sound daunting, the effort is worth it. After all, who wouldn't want a chance at a longer, happier, and healthier life? By observing and learning from Blue Zones around the world, we gain valuable insights into the true art of living well.

Now the challenge lies with you. Go out and create your own Blue Zone. Delve into the healthy, mindful, and communal ways of living that these areas exemplify. A longer, healthier, more fulfilling life is within your reach. You simply need to extend your hand and grasp it.

Challenges and Considerations

Despite the numerous case studies and substantial evidence from the Blue Zones regarding increased longevity, it's important to understand that implementing these practices into your own life isn't a one-size-fits-all solution. You'll face challenges and considerations that need careful thought and planning.

First and foremost, adhering to the dietary habits of a traditional Sardinian may not be practical or feasible for many people. Sardinians thrive on a diet rich in whole foods, fruits, vegetables, lean proteins, and whole grains, largely cultivated from their lands. In many modern societies, access to such fresh, organic and locally-sourced foods can be both costly and challenging to find.

Also, many cultures across the world have dietary practices and food preferences deeply ingrained in their lifestyle and traditions. Adopting a Mediterranean-style diet, despite its proven health benefits, may conflict with established eating patterns, making it a difficult lifestyle modification to implement and sustain in the long run.

Additionally, the role of physical activity in Sardinian society stems from daily farming, herding, and routine manual chores. In contrast, much of the urban world is shifting towards sedentary work styles and automation. Mimicking the kind of constant, low-intensity physical activity Sardinians engage in may not be feasible for those living in environments lacking this kind of active lifestyle infrastructure.

Navigating socio-cultural differences is another hurdle. The strong sense of community, togetherness, and emphasis on close-knit family units is at the heart of Sardinian culture. In many parts of the world, societal structures are notably different, with a huge emphasis on individualism. Transitioning from an individualistic philosophy to a community-centric one could pose a significant cultural challenge.

Moreover, the Sardinians' emphasis on appreciating life's simple pleasures, long-term contentment, and stress management techniques are vastly different from the "go-go-go" mentality often observed in the current societal mindset. It might be challenging to slow down, reflect, and enjoy living in the moment in the constant pursuit of achievement, wealth, and outward success, which is common in many modern societies.

Beyond these practical considerations, there's also the matter of genetics playing a role in longevity. While the environment and lifestyle have substantial impacts, the genetic makeups of these long-living individuals may contain specific variants that contribute to their longevity. Not everyone may be biologically equipped with similar genetic advantages.

Even the climate of Sardinia is not easily replicated. The Mediterranean climate, with its warm summers and mild winters, plays a role in outdoor activity level, food planting and harvesting cycles, and even mood and psychological well-being.

When trying to adopt the practices of the Sardinian people, we must bear in mind that they have evolved these practices over many generations, in harmony with their environment and their cultural beliefs. It's not as simple as picking and choosing certain elements and expecting them to work the same independently.

However, this is not to discourage you from your quest in applying Sardinian wisdom to your life. Yes, the transitions may seem challenging, but the aim is to find a balance, to seek inspiration, and to adapt as much as possible from the Blue Zone's lifestyle that fits your own local and cultural context.

The key to this approach lies in personalization: understanding your circumstances, evaluating the practicality of implementing changes, and then adapting the elements that are doable and sustainable for you. It's about making incremental changes, not wholesale ones.

Though the challenges of merging another culture's ways into your lifestyle are real, remember that the journey to longevity is much like Sardinia's own: not a sudden sprint, but a continual, steady journey of many steps, in tune with the rhythms of nature and society.

Whatever challenges one might face in attempting to apply the lessons of the Blue Zones, it's crucial to remember that the underlying principles - whole food diets, physical activity, community engagement, and stress reduction - have universal relevance and can be adapted to most situations in some form or another.

Wisdom from the elders of Sardinia, this Blue Zone island, doesn't aim to offer a magical elixir of life, but rather inspires us to review, revisit and reinvent our lifestyles in pursuit of healthier, more contented, and hopefully, longer lives.

Chapter 10: Conclusion - A Legacy of Longevity

In the all-encompassing journey through the land of centenarians, the collective wisdom of Sardinia unravels a fascinating correlation between lifestyle factors and remarkable longevity. The harmonious balance between the Sardinian diet, family ties, physical activity, emotional wellness, and healthcare practices casts a bountiful landscape rich with vital lessons for healthier living. Their deeply ingrained culture of community cooperation, active living, and serene spirituality extends beyond Sardinia, resonating within other global blue zones. Implementing these insights into our own lives, although challenging, can set us on a path towards our own blue zone, fostering a legacy of prolonged vitality and health. Excitingly, there is still terrain to be explored when it comes to longevity research, and the tantalizing prospect of future endeavors in this realm of study remains. But, as we conclude, it's evident that the enduring legacy of Sardinia is its gift to humanity; an insightful revelation on the magic of longevity.

Summary of Findings

Our exploration into the enigmatic longevity of Sardinia's Blue Zones presents intriguing insights. Central to the Sardinians' prolonged lifespan is their dietary culture, deeply ingrained societal norms, routines and physical activities, emotional and spiritual wellness practices, and unique healthcare methods. Collectively, these factors foster an environment conducive to health, well-being, and longevity.

The geographical and demographical characteristics of Sardinia play an integral role in their longevity. The island's isolated location contributes significantly, resulting in dietary practices that revolve around locally sourced ingredients. The Sardinian diet is a remarkable blend of Mediterranean influences, with a strong reliance on whole foods, plant-based nutrition, sea-based protein sources, and moderate wine consumption.

Physical activities and work also contribute to their well-being. Sardinians tend to have physically demanding daily routines involving manual labor, cultivations, and traditional craftsmanship. This regular, moderate physical exertion inadvertently promotes fitness and health, reducing the risk of cardiovascular and metabolic diseases.

Family and communal bonds are notably robust in Sardinian society. The social structure in Sardinia is rooted in familial ties, community engagement, and mutual support. This emotionally supportive environment contributes to mental health, reducing stress levels, and promoting happiness, which unquestionably positively impact longevity in this region.

Another crucial aspect of the Sardinian lifestyle is the emphasis on emotional and spiritual wellness. Traditional beliefs and practices are conserved and respected. The Sardinians demonstrate a profound sense of mindfulness and contentment, further promoting emotional balance and overall health.

The healthcare practices in Sardinia are unique and richly integrated, combining conventional medical treatments with preventive measures. Conventional healthcare is coupled with the belief in restorative properties of natural ingredients and traditional, often home-based, remedies. In this way, health is treated not merely as a lack of illness but as holistic well-being.

The stories shared by Sardinian centenarians provided valuable personal perspectives on longevity. Their wisdom and life lessons highlighted the importance of respecting seasoned traditions, eating local, maintaining a balanced life laden with physical activities, and preserving strong social connections.

The comparison with other global Blue Zones further emphasized common elements found in areas known for notable longevity: wholesome eating, active living, effective healthcare, and strong community ties. Yet, each Blue Zone has unique adaptations of these elements, reflecting their regional influences.

The practical application of Sardinian wisdom suggests a paradigm shift in our approach to health and longevity. The need to create our own Blue Zone involves embracing an active lifestyle, eating a balanced diet, nurturing social connections, and fostering emotional and spiritual wellness. This entails both simple adjustments and significant changes, each person and community facing distinct challenges dictated by their circumstances.

The legacy of Sardinian longevity provides us not just with fascinating anecdotes of centenarians but also with a roadmap to healthier and longer living. It encourages embracing a locally centric dietary routine, fostering physically active lifestyles, celebrating communal bonds, and encapsulating holistic healthcare practices.

In summary, the key to Sardinians' remarkable lifespan lies in the dynamic integration of a healthy diet, physical activities, strong social and familial ties, emotional balance, spiritual wellness, and effective healthcare. These aspects are not addressed separately, but rather intertwined and mutually reinforcing, creating an environment that fosters well-being and longevity.

Finally, the findings also highlight the paramount importance of adaptation. There is no universally applicable, "one-size-fits-all" longevity formula. Each Blue Zone has tailored these elements to fit their cultural and regional contexts. Hence, it is evident that creating our own Blue Zone would need a certain level of customization to our unique circumstances while maintaining the core principles of health and longevity derived from Sardinian wisdom.

This journey into the heart of Sardinia's Blue Zones leaves us with profound insights and an inspired perspective on living a long, healthy, and fulfilling life. It's about creating a harmonious fusion of dietary, physical, social, emotional, and spiritual aspects that promote overall well-being. This isn't merely about chronological age but embracing a lifestyle that nurtures holistically healthy, fulfilled, and extended lives.

With future research focusing on other Blue Zones around the world, we can continue to explore and learn from the various paths that lead to longevity. It will provide a richer understanding of the intricate factors influencing longevity and how to successfully implement these lessons into our lives.

Reflections on the Journey

The narrative of Sardinia's remarkable longevity is akin to an ageless and vibrant tapestry, woven with stories of individuals who have experienced a century of living, the historical context that shaped their existence, and the crucial elements that contributed to their extraordinary lifespans. Our exploration of this mystifying Blue Zone has been an enlightening journey, painting a fascinating picture of a lifestyle anchored in balanced nutrition, strong social ties, significant physical activity, emotional wellness, and an integrative healthcare approach.

Reflecting on the Sardinian diet, it's evident that what these centenarians consume daily is less about 'dieting' and more about a holistic lifestyle, infused with local, nutrient-rich ingredients. Their diets provide an excellent example of how Mediterranean influences, coupled with local produce and traditional cooking methods, result in a wholesome, balanced dietary regimen that not only satiates but also sustains. Their love for beans, whole grains, fruits, and vegetables, with modest indulgence in health-promoting wine and locally cured meat, sets a precedent for people worldwide who seek long, healthy lives.

The notion of community, deeply ingrained in Sardinian society, is another factor that transcends their cultural façade. Observing centuries-old traditions, their close-knit family structures and robust social ties serve as an effective support network—an antidote to modern loneliness and isolation. The sense of belonging they derive from their communities, engaging in regular social interactions, undoubtedly contributes significantly to their mental health resilience and overall well-being.

The engagement of their bodies in rigorous, daily physical activity invariably captured attention, highlighting the vitality of regular exercise and active living. From light, incidental exercise, like walking, to strenuous activities involved in herding, farming, and house chores, these centenarians demonstrate that physical activity does not need to be structured or mundane; it can merely be an integral part of daily routines and life.

Equally vital is the often-underestimated realm of emotional and spiritual wellness that beautifully coexists with the physical aspect of their lives. Their traditional beliefs and practices, coupled with their mindfulness and contented mindset, form an effective coping mechanism against emotional upheavals and stress, contributing immensely to their extended lifespans.

Our exploration also extended to the understanding of Sardinian healthcare practices, which interestingly correlate with their cultural beliefs and traditions. Their integrative health approach, which emphasizes prevention and holistic care, appears not only robust but highly efficacious, signifying the need for similar practices worldwide.

Listening to the stories of Sardinian elders added profoundness to this entire exploration. Their wisdom, experiences, and personal perspectives on longevity unravel the life lessons that seem to create not only their multi-decade existence but also the true richness of their lives. Their unique ability to savor life's simplicity and carry forward a legacy of wisdom is truly remarkable.

Extending our knowledge beyond Sardinia to other global blue zones, it becomes apparent that universally, across all blue zones, some similar patterns have emerged. Chief among these are a healthy diet, community engagement, regular physical exercises, balanced emotional health, and integrative health practices. Yet, each blue zone's unique cultural context adds a distinct flavor to the longevity recipe, offering vast possibilities for global health improvement.

Applying the Sardinian wisdom gleaned through this journey and translating it to our personal lives might seem challenging. However, practical steps towards healthier living, in congruence with your cultural and contextual realities, can gradually create your own blue zone. I urge you to strive to incorporate these lessons in your life. If obstacles appear, apprehend, and address them—it's a journey worth undertaking!

In conclusion, our exploration of Sardinian longevity has been an enlightening amalgamation of scientific scrutiny, journalistic curiosity, and a profound respect for the unique cultural tapestry that is the essence of Sardinian life. This journey has shed light on the manifold ways we can enrich our lives with healthier dietary choices, meaningful social interactions, physical activities, emotional balance, and conscious pursuit of happiness.

Looking ahead, there's undoubtedly a scope for more research—studies that delve deeper into the genetics of Sardinians, food studies that highlight the nutritional profile of the traditional diet, and sociological studies that explore the effect of the Sardinian way of life on overall human health. This unraveled mystery of Sardinian longevity serves as a beacon for future endeavors, illuminating the path towards globally viable and adaptable lifestyle strategies conducive to long, healthy, and fulfilling lives. To longevity and beyond!

Future Research and Endeavors

As we draw the curtains on this engaging narrative on Sardinian longevity, it's essential to note that the world of science and wellness invariably move forward. Human comprehension of longevity's secrets hidden in these blue zones stays a work-in-progress, with far more unanswered questions than firm conclusions.

Sardinia undoubtedly holds important keys to understanding longevity, but it is merely one piece of the puzzle. Future investigations can explore other geographical blue zones to identify their unique practices, regional diets, and community structures, making the concept of human longevity more understandable.

Additionally, within Sardinia itself, there are potential undiscovered sub-regions with unique characteristics contributing to their inhabitants' impressive lifespan. While we have managed to add some color to the once-cloudy picture of Sardinia's longevity, entirely cracking the Sardinian enigma demands more targeted research focused on isolating specific variables.

Another promising direction for future inquiries lies in genetics. Although we have discussed the general influence of genetics on longevity in Sardinia, we still have limited understanding of the specific genes involved. Future genetic investigations into these unique populations may unlock the doors to potential natural genetic enhancements or interventions.

The role of diet and nutrition can't be stressed enough. While we've dipped into the Mediterranean influences and local ingredients of Sardinian cuisine, a deeper exploration of micro-ingredients with potential health benefits opens up an exciting field for future research.

What about the mind-body connection and the spiritual practices observed in Sardinia? Unraveling the specific psychological pathways that contribute to longevity and wellness remains a stimulating challenge for the scientific community. The integration of these traditional practices with modern healthcare models could provide innovative ways to maintain mental and physical health.

Family bonds and social ties appear as another crucial aspect contributing to Sardinian longevity. Therefore, a scientific inquiry excavating deeper into the nature of these social dynamics – how they form, evolve, and impact wellness – also presents itself as an exciting research avenue. It can stimulate dialogues around how modern societies globally can nurture, protect, and enrich these networks.

Indeed, the importance of physical activity in achieving longevity is evident in the Sardinian lifestyle. But specifying what kind of activity, its frequency and intensity, and its unique impacts compared to other types of exercises could elucidate the link between physical activity and health span even further.

Diving into the cultural and historical aspects of longevity in Sardinia may also yield fascinating insights. It would be worthwhile to investigate how these traditions have endured and adapted over time and their nuanced interplay with genetic, physical, and dietary factors.

Exploring the relationship between income, education, and longevity will also prove insightful. How do these socio-economic factors shape the contours of longevity in Sardinia and other blue zones? Do they magnify or diminish other influences on lifespan? Here, the interplay of social determinants of health and longevity offers fertile ground for research.

And what about other forms of wellness—not only physical, but emotional, spiritual, and mental? Future studies can shine a light on the impact of various forms of wellbeing on longevity, further enriching our understanding of how to live not just long, but well.

Lastly, medical models and preventive measures in Sardinian society could provide fresh ways to think about healthcare elsewhere. Mapping these local practices onto more extensive healthcare systems may lead to novel, integrative strategies for disease prevention and health promotion.

The road to unlocking the secrets of human longevity is long and winding, awash with less-travelled paths begging exploration. These offer exciting and promising directions for future inquiries to further demystify the blue zones of the world.

In essence, our journey into the heart of Sardinia and its unique longevity ecosystem is just the beginning—a stepping stone onto a broader platform of understanding this compelling subject. Here's to the future research and endeavors, as we all share the common goal of comprehending and, hopefully, achieving the secret to a longer, healthier life.

Appendix A: Appendices

This appendix seeks to provide supplementary material to the concepts and theories that have been addressed throughout this book. It serves as an enriching resource, allowing the reader to delve deeper into the subject of longevity in Blue Zones, with a specific reflection on Sardinia. It's divided into three sections: Additional Recipes, Research Methodologies, and Recommended Reading and Resources.

Additional Recipes

We've talked extensively about the Mediterranean diet and the key role it plays in Sardinian longevity. To enable you to embrace this lifestyle more fully, we're providing some extra traditional Sardinian recipes that have passed down over the generations. Amping up your meals on these nutritious recipes might just increase your chances of joining the centenarian club.

Research Methodologies

Throughout this book, we've discussed various scientific research and studies to better understand the enigmatic longevity in Sardinia. But if you're interested in the nuts and bolts of the research process itself, we've included a section on the methodologies used in these studies. We've painstakingly teased out the result to provide factually accurate information, keeping in line with our journalistic approach to make the research process transparent to our readers. Approaches featured here include qualitative and quantitative methods from in-depth interviews to statistical analyses.

Recommended Reading and Resources

If you're still hungry for more knowledge, we got you covered. We've listed out numerous books, scholarly articles, documentaries, and websites that delve into the topic of longevity, Blue Zones, and Sardinian culture more broadly. These resources are vetted, credible and focus on three primary areas: cultural studies, dietary habits, and explorations of centenarian lifestyle. We believe this will give you a comprehensive understanding, bringing you a step closer to actualizing a Blue Zone lifestyle in your environment.

Conclusion

Bearing in mind the old saying, "Knowledge is power," we hope that this appendix enlightens you further on the paths to healthier, more sustainable living. Rooted in the practices of the longest-living individuals in Sardinia, these principles are not only fascinating but also potently effective. Here's to your journey toward a longer, healthier life!

Additional Recipes: The Sardinian diet, rich in foods directly harvested from the land and sea, plays a pivotal role in facilitating the longevity of Sardinian people. Yet, the diet is not all about consuming certain ingredients; it also emphasizes the manner in which dishes are lovingly prepared and shared amongst the community. This exploration extends beyond the recipes detailed in Chapter 2, showcasing additional Sardinian recipes intrinsic to the island's food culture and capable of supporting a long and healthy life.

Sardinian Minestrone: This warming soup stew stands as a testament to the island's love of legumes and vegetables. Key ingredients include fava beans, chickpeas, potatoes, and an assortment of locally cultivated vegetables. What makes this dish truly Sardinian is the use of fregula, small round balls of semolina dough that provide a satisfying texture to the soup.

Ingredients:

- Fava beans

- Chickpeas

- Potatoes

- Assortment of vegetables

- Fregula

Panada: This savory pie finds its place in nearly every Sardinian celebration, encapsulating the spirit of hearty meals and family togetherness. The traditional Panada is packed with eel, potatoes, and onions, although variations may include lamb, artichokes, or peas. The golden, flaky crust seals in robust flavors, making it a one-dish wonder.

Ingredients:

- Eel or Lamb

- Potatoes

- Onions

- Artichokes

- Peas

Dolce di Noci (Walnut Sweets): These sweet, crumbly delights translate the island's abundance of walnuts into a treasured dessert. Prepared with a combination of walnuts, honey, and lemon zest, it delivers a perfectly balanced palate of sweetness, tartness, and nuttiness. Believed to contribute to brain health, these walnut sweets are a nutritious end to any meal.

Ingredients:

- Walnuts

- Honey

- Lemon zest

The beauty of Sardinian cuisine lies in its simplicity, putting a spotlight on the island's quality ingredients. Each of these recipes, when made with fresh, local, and seasonal produce, encapsulate the magic of Sardinian eating habits - a mixture of healthy ingredients, mindful preparation, and sharing with loved ones.

As you experiment with these recipes, allow the flavors to transport you to Sardinian blue-zone kitchens, infusing your wellness journey with an additional layer of authenticity. More importantly, endeavor to infuse the spirit of community and joy into your meals, turning every dining occasion into a celebration of health and longevity.

Research Methodologies To unearth the secret behind Sardinian longevity, a fusion of qualitative and quantitative research methodologies were employed to explore the factors that contribute to the inhabitants' long and healthy lives. Detailed attention was paid to the local diet, lifestyle factors and community connections, utilizing modern scientific tools alongside traditional anthropological exploration.

Among the quantitative techniques, epidemiological methods, nutritional analyses, and physical examinations were employed. These empirical tools allowed us to construct a database that reflects on the health conditions and lifestyle habits in Sardinia. Epidemiological studies provided the opportunity to compare and contrast the rate of chronic diseases and causes of death with other regions in the world, while nutritional analyses offered valuable insights into the dietary patterns within this blue zone.

Besides these scientific methodologies, a slew of qualitative methods, like interviews with centenarians, comprehensive document studies, and participatory observation, offered invaluable insights. Stories, wisdom, and life lessons from the elders, their personal perspectives on longevity, were extracted through these interviews.

Participatory observation methodologies were, particularly, exciting as it provided a first-hand experience of the Sardinian way of life. By living amidst them, adopting their schedule, and participating in their day-to-day activities, we collected important data on the local diet, relationships, community activities, and general lifestyle habits. This approach gave a unique insight into the sociocultural context in which Sardinians are living their elongated and wholesome lives.

Documentary studies also played a pivotal role, as they delve into the historical records, demographical data, healthcare practices, and every fine detail that paints the whole picture of Sardinia's place in the longevity landscape. This incorporated a thorough review of surveys, government reports, medical records, and related artifacts.

These combined research methodologies ensured an embodied understanding of the Sardinian lifestyle and provided a breadth of insight into how the people in these blue zones live. It was an interplay between observed lifestyle data and interpreted experiences meaningfully combined to create a robust framework of Sardinian longevity.

Recommended Reading and Resources. The journey of understanding the longevity mystery of Sardinia's Blue Zone doesn't stop after the last page of this book. There are numerous resources that you can delve into to continue expanding your knowledge.

Let's start with the cornerstone resource, *The Blue Zones: Lessons for Living Longer From the People Who've Lived the Longest* by Dan Buettner. Buettner's research and collaboration with National Geographic and longevity experts led to identifying five "Blue Zones" around the world, including Sardinia. His book thoroughly explores lifestyles in these zones and offers significant insights into their longevity practices.

Ikigai: The Japanese Secret to a Long and Happy Life by Héctor García and Francesc Miralles offers an insightful dive into a concept that can be called the Japanese equivalent of Sardinia's shepherding tradition, which certainly contributes to long life. The book explores the notion of *Ikigai*, linking one's passion, mission, profession, and vocation, which is central to the life of the people of Okinawa, another famed Blue Zone.

Another significant book is *Healthy at 100* by John Robbins. Being an environmentalist, his reflections on diet, environment, lifestyle, and their connection to longevity are compelling. This book particularly sheds light on life-extending practices in a few societies worldwide.

For a broader perspective that goes beyond the Mediterranean, you can't miss *The China Study* by T. Colin Campbell and Thomas M. Campbell II. It's a comprehensive review of the relationship between diet and disease, offering valuable insights about food, health, and longevity.

Online Resources

Longevity and Blue Zones aren't merely limited to books. Several websites and online platforms provide valuable resources:

- *The Blue Zones* website provides various articles, interviews, recipes, and lifestyle tips drawing from the world's five original Blue Zones.

- *Longevity* Research Institute at Oxford sheds light on current research projects and findings to those interested in the scientific side of longevity.

- *The Okinawa Centenarian Study* website offers a wealth of information on the study that's been running for close to half a century, focusing on the extraordinary elders of Okinawa, Japan.

Our journey into the mystery of the Blue Zones is fascinating, with research and resources continuously growing. By exploring these recommended readings and resources, your understanding and appreciation of the role that lifestyle, diet, relationships, physical and emotional wellness play in our longevity is bound to deepen. As you carve your own path into healthier and perhaps longer living, remember the lessons from Sardinia and let them guide you.